ALZHEIM.
DISEASE
QUESTIONS AND ANSWERS

SECOND EDITION

PAUL S AISEN, MD
Department of Neurology, Georgetown University Medical Center

DEBORAH B MARIN, MD
Department of Psychiatry, Mount Sinai Medical Center

KENNETH L DAVIS, MD
Department of Psychiatry, Mount Sinai Medical Center

JENNIFER HOBLYN, MD
Department of Psychiatry, Mount Sinai Medical Center

ELIZABETH FINE, MSW, CSW
Department of Geriatrics & Adult Development, Mount Sinai Medical Center

JAY J SANGERMAN, ESQ
Jay J Sangerman & Associates, Attorneys at Law, New York City, New York

merit
PUBLISHING
INTERNATIONAL

7/99

merit
PUBLISHING
INTERNATIONAL

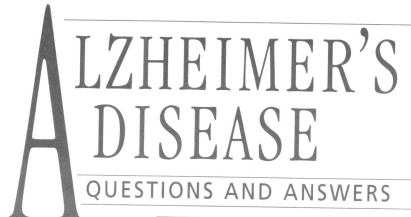

ALZHEIMER'S DISEASE

QUESTIONS AND ANSWERS

SECOND EDITION

MERIT PUBLISHING INTERNATIONAL

European address:
35 Winchester Street
Basingstoke
Hampshire RG21 7EE
England

North American address:
8260 NW 49th Manor
Pine Grove, Coral Springs
Florida 33067
U.S.A.

ISBN 1 873413 52 1

PAUL S AISEN

DEBORAH B MARIN

KENNETH L DAVIS

m*e*rit
PUBLISHING
INTERNATIONAL

ALZHEIMER'S DISEASE

PREFACE

When Alzheimer's disease is raised as a diagnostic consideration, patients and their families suddenly confront the staggering ramifications of this slowly but relentlessly progressive and ultimately devastating condition. The issues that must be addressed are too many and too complex to be covered in routine sessions with healthcare providers; the difficulty is usually compounded by emotional upheaval which interferes with effective communication. In addition, the primary care physicians who first consider the diagnosis may not be fully informed in all areas of this rapidly changing field.

Our intention in preparing this book was to raise the pertinent questions and provide clear and concise answers. We have tried to provide explanations understandable to non-clinicians, but also to explore the issues in sufficient depth to be useful to healthcare professionals, including physicians.

Since publication of the first edition of this book, there has been steady progress in basic and clinical research related to Alzheimer's disease. Our understanding of the molecular and cellular changes that occur in the brain continues to advance. Physicians are better able to treat the cognitive and behavioral manifestations. But perhaps most important, effective treatment to slow the disease process may not be far off. This book has been extensively revised to reflect the changing field, including the addition of a chapter describing research into disease-modifying therapies. The major scientific papers published in recent years have been added to the reference list. It is our hope that this edition captures the excitement and optimism of current research into Alzheimer's disease.

CONTENTS

ALZHEIMER'S DISEASE

Is aluminum a risk factor for Alzheimer's disease?

Is zinc a risk factor for Alzheimer's disease?

What is the relationship between Down syndrome and Alzheimer's disease?

Are there any factors that may decrease the risk for Alzheimer's disease?

Is estrogen protective against Alzheimer's disease?

Does aspirin or ibuprofen protect against Alzheimer's disease?

Can antioxidants, and even the antioxidant vitamins, diminish the likelihood of Alzheimer's disease?

6. **What are the clinical manifestations of Alzheimer's disease? 53**
Deborah B. Marin and Jennifer Hoblyn

What are the symptoms of Alzheimer's disease?

What changes in memory occur in Alzheimer's disease?

How does Alzheimer's disease affect one's orientation?

How is language affected in Alzheimer's disease?

How are problem solving and judgment affected in Alzheimer's disease?

What impact does Alzheimer's disease have on an individual's involvement in the community?

What about driving?

How does Alzheimer's disease affect personal care and grooming?

What behavioral changes occur in Alzheimer's disease?

What mood changes occur in Alzheimer's disease?

What personality changes occur in Alzheimer's disease?

What perceptual changes occur in Alzheimer's disease?

Does agitation occur in Alzheimer's disease?

What is the course of Alzheimer's disease symptoms?

Who covers the cost of a nursing home?

How does one make the home safe for the Alzheimer's disease patient?

How should one communicate with an Alzheimer's patient?

What activities are recommended with Alzheimer's disease patients?

Is Alzheimer's disease treatable?

What can be done to improve a patient's memory?

What is an appropriate expectation for the cognitive effects of cholinesterase inhibitors?

Why does it take so long to reach these upper doses of tacrine?

How do donepezil and tacrine compare?

Are other drugs besides donepezil and tacrine in development?

Are there other approaches to increased cholinergic activity?

Are there drugs that may stop the progression of Alzheimer's disease?

If a drug is developed to slow the progression of Alzheimer's disease, when should treatment begin?

What is the theory behind the use of antioxidants to treat Alzheimer's disease?

What is the theory behind the studies of anti-inflammatory treatments for Alzheimer's disease?

Is Alzheimer's disease an inflammatory disease?

If the inflammatory theory is true, will any anti-inflammatory drug work?

Which anti-inflammatory drugs show the greatest promise?

What is the status of anti-inflammatory drug trials?

Since so much is written about anti-inflammatory and antioxidant agents, should everyone take ibuprofen and vitamins to prevent Alzheimer's disease?

What is the evidence that estrogen will be useful in the treatment of Alzheimer's disease?

Is there any medication that can prevent the deposition of amyloid in the brain?

What other strategies are being pursued to slow the course of Alzheimer's disease?

If a drug is developed that can slow the course of Alzheimer's disease, will symptomatic treatment still be necessary?

How do we avoid quackery?

How can the non-cognitive symptoms of Alzheimer's disease be treated?

What is the role of antipsychotic medication in Alzheimer's disease?

Are there advantages to new, recently developed antipsychotic medications?

What are the alternatives to antipsychotic medications in the treatment of behavioral disturbances in Alzheimer's disease?

Are there special considerations in the treatment of depression in patients with Alzheimer's disease?

Can sedatives be used safely?

What is the story with melatonin?

When else does a power-of-attorney become terminated?

Does a power-of-attorney ever become irrevocable?

How many agents can there be in a power-of-attorney?

If there are multiple agents, must they act together or can they have separate and equal authority?

In addition to a general power-of-attorney, should the principal have powers-of-attorney at individual financial institutions?

How many original powers-of-attorney should the principal execute?

Need the principal keep powers-of-attorney current?

Can the agent take or gift to others the principal's property?

Are standard forms available for powers-of-attorney?

What problems should be considered prior to executing a power-of-attorney?

TRUST AGREEMENT

What is a "trust?"

Are there any rules for the operation of the trust?

What are some of the provisions which might be included in the trust agreement?

Can a trust be amended or revoked?

Who can be a trustee?

What mental capacity is required for the formation of a trust?

If a person has a trust, need s/he also have a last will and testament?

What are the disadvantages of a trust?

What are the advantages of a trust?

Does a trust require the trustee to render an annual accounting?

JOINT ACCOUNTS

What are joint accounts?

Can joint accounts be used for asset management?

How does a joint account affect an estate plan?

How does a joint account affect estate tax planning?

What are the advantages of jointly held property?

Can either joint tenant withdraw funds from a joint account or manage the property within the joint account?

What is the disadvantage of jointly held assets?

PLANNING FOR FUTURE MEDICAL DECISION-MAKING

What kind of planning should be done for the Alzheimer's patient in regard to future medical decision-making?

What is a Living Will?

What problems can be encountered with a Living Will?

Can an individual appoint an agent to make medical decisions when the individual cannot communicate his/her preferences?

Is the appointment of an agent in one state valid in other states?

What mental capacity is required to appoint an agent to make medical decisions?

What considerations should be taken prior to the execution of a living will or appointment of an agent?

Who should be the agent?

How many agents can there be?

Can the agent make any medical decision for the principal?

Should a person execute both a living will and a document appointing an agent?

Can there be surrogate decision-making in the absence of an advance directive?

ALZHEIMER'S DISEASE

If an individual has both a power-of-attorney and an advance medical directive, will all decisions be able to be made in the event of incapacity?

Is a doctor's letter useful to have in the patient's file as to mental capacity?

How is a guardian appointed?

What powers is the guardian given?

Who makes the determination of mental capacity?

What can medical providers do to protect themselves when treating patients of questionable mental capacity?

Is it safe for medical providers to make determinations of mental capacity for the execution of legal documents?

III. PAYING FOR LONG-TERM CARE

Is there insurance available to cover nursing home care?

If I qualify, what should I look for in long-term insurance?

Do long-term care policies cover care at home?

Where do I receive information about long-term care insurance?

Does Medicare pay for nursing home care?

What are the criteria for Medicare payment for the nursing home stay?

When will I know if Medicare will cover my nursing home stay?

Will Medicare pay for homecare?

Can life insurance be used to pay for long-term care?

Will Medicaid pay for long-term care in a nursing home?

Does the Alzheimer's patient need to be poor to qualify for Medicaid?

Can the Alzheimer's patient divest him/herself of assets after admission to a nursing home?

Does one require special advice as to divestment of assets?

Can an advanced Alzheimer's patient who does not have the capacity to participate in financial decision-making be divested of assets?

Where can one go for advice about planning for long-term care?

Are there any other sources of payment to the Alzheimer's patient that should be considered?

What if the Alzheimer's patient does not qualify for Social Security Disability payments. Are there other sources of funds available?

ALZHEIMER'S DISEASE

CHAPTER 1

WHAT IS ALZHEIMER'S DISEASE?

What is meant by the term?

Alzheimer's disease is an illness that causes progressive cognitive impairment. It is a treatable, but not yet curable disease. Memory, particularly the capacity to retain new information, is most prominently affected. However other cognitive functions, including orientation, language, judgment, social functioning and the ability to perform motor tasks (praxis), also decline as the disease progresses. Changes in brain tissue, specifically the formation of amyloid plaques and neurofibrillary tangles and the loss of brain cells, lead to the impairment of these brain functions. The illness is strongly associated with age; it is uncommon before age 50, but may affect as many as half of all people who live into their 90s.

How is it related to normal aging? to senility? to simple forgetfulness?

Alzheimer's disease was first described by the pathologist Alois Alzheimer in the early years of this century. During the decades since the original report, there has been much confusion and debate regarding terminology, and the relationship of this illness to normal aging. Part of the difficulty stems from the fact that the microscopic changes seen in the brains of patients with Alzheimer's disease are also found in the brains of unaffected elderly people; the difference lies in quantity and distribution of changes.

Senility, defined by dictionaries as a deterioration in physical or mental function as a result of old age, is not a medical term. Nonetheless, until recently it was common to refer to Alzheimer's disease in relatively young patients as "presenile dementia," and Alzheimer's disease in older individuals as "senile dementia" or "Senile Dementia of the Alzheimer Type." These terms have now been largely abandoned.

Dementia is the medical term for global cognitive dysfunction. Dementia may occur in many different diseases, including cerebrovascular disease

ALZHEIMER'S DISEASE

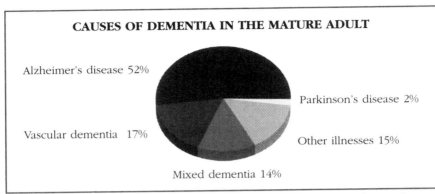

CAUSES OF DEMENTIA IN THE MATURE ADULT

Alzheimer's disease 52%

Parkinson's disease 2%

Vascular dementia 17%

Other illnesses 15%

Mixed dementia 14%

Figure 1.1 *Demonstrates the most common causes of memory disorders in the mature adult. Alzheimer's disease and vascular dementia account for the majority of dementias. Mixed dimentia refers to a dementia that includes both Alzheimer's disease and vascular dementia.*

(strokes), alcoholism and the Acquired Immune Deficiency Syndrome. As illustrated in Figure 1.1, Alzheimer's disease is the most common cause of dementia worldwide, comprising over 50% of cases. Most of the remaining cases can be attributed to stroke (vascular dementia), or a combination of stroke plus Alzheimer's disease (mixed dementia).

There are changes in memory and other cognitive functions that occur as a natural consequence of aging. Practically, such changes can be distinguished from dementia on the basis of functional significance. In dementia, cognitive decline results in loss of function, that is, decline in ability to manage the responsibilities of home and work, social activities, or even activities of daily living. Impairment in memory is necessary, but not sufficient for a diagnosis of dementia; decline in at least one other area of cognitive functioning is necessary. To be diagnostic, these impairments must cause difficulty in social, occupational, or day to day functioning. Chapter 6 reviews the symptoms of dementia in greater detail.

In the past decade or so, experts in this field have reached a consensus that Alzheimer's disease is in fact a disease, in which degeneration of brain cells results from one or more genetic and/or environmental factors. Much effort is now devoted to the identification of remediable factors that contribute to the loss of brain function in Alzheimer's disease. Most experts do not believe that dementia is an invariable consequence of aging. There is optimism that research will uncover interventions that will delay or prevent the occurrence and progression of the symptoms of Alzheimer's disease.

How is the diagnosis made?

At the present time, a definitive diagnosis of Alzheimer's disease can only be made after careful examination of brain tissue. Such an examination can only occur with tissue obtained after death at autopsy, or by biopsy (sampling) of brain tissue while the patient is living. Brain biopsy is rarely performed. Therefore, a definitive diagnosis of Alzheimer's disease is rarely possible before death.

When physicians make the diagnosis of Alzheimer's disease, they are in fact indicating that a patient meets the clinical criteria for the diagnosis of probable Alzheimer's disease. There are two formal sets of criteria for this diagnosis that physicians frequently refer to: the *Diagnostic and Statistical Manual of Mental Disorders, Fourth Edition* (DSM-IV)(Figure 1.2), and the

---

DIAGNOSTIC CRITERIA FOR
DEMENTIA OF THE ALZHEIMER'S TYPE*

A. The development of multiple cognitive deficits manifested by both:

1. memory impairment, and

2. one (or more) of the following cognitive disturbances:
   a. aphasia (language disturbance)
   b. apraxia (impaired ability to carry out motor activities despite intact motor function)
   c. agnosia (failure to recognize or identify objects despite intact sensory function)
   d. disturbance in executive functioning (i.e. planning, organization, sequencing, abstracting)

B. The congitive deficits in Criteria A1 and A2 each cause significant impairment in social or occupational functioning and represent a significant decline from a previous level of functioning

C. The course is characterized by gradual onset and continuing cognitive decline

D. The cognitive deficits in Criteria A1 and A2 are not due to any other medical conditions that causes progressive deficits in memory and cognition

---

Figure 1.2 *Lists the criteria for Alzheimer's disease*. *Adapted from 'The Diagnostic and Statistical Manual of Mental Disorders', 4th edition.*

ALZHEIMER'S DISEASE

National Institute of Neurological and Communicative Disorders, Stroke, Alzheimer's Disease, and Related Disorders Association (NINCDS-ADRDA) criteria. The two sets of criteria are comparable. Both of these published guidelines require a diagnosis of progressive dementia, along with the exclusion of other possible explanations for the dementia. Thus, it is often said that Alzheimer's disease is a diagnosis of exclusion.

The reported accuracy of the clinical diagnosis of probable Alzheimer's disease (compared with the ultimate post-mortem diagnosis) varies, but is roughly 85-90% with a comprehensive evaluation. Use of the apolipoprotein E genetic test (see chapter 4) can improve the accuracy of diagnosis by about 5%.

What is the standard work-up?

When a physician makes any medical diagnosis, he/she obtains a history, performs an examination, obtains any necessary tests, then synthesizes all of the information (see Figure 1.3). Most often, the history is obtained from the patient seeking medical advice. In the evaluation of memory impairment, however, it may not be possible to obtain reliable information from the patient; family members and others close to the patient are typically the primary source of the medical history.

Just as with the majority of medical illnesses, the most important component of the evaluation of a person with possible Alzheimer's disease is an accurate history. From the detailed history, the clinician judges whether functionally significant cognitive decline has occurred, and may uncover possible causes of brain dysfunction (e.g. chronic alcohol use).

EVALUATION OF A PATIENT WITH DEMENTIA

◆ A clinical history from the patient and an informant, usually a family member

◆ Physical examination

◆ Testing of memory and other cognitive functions

◆ Labs: blood counts, chemistries, B-12, level, thyroid function test, syphilis test

◆ Brain imaging: CT scan or MRI scan

Figure 1.3 *Lists the components of a comprehensive evaluation of an individual who presents with cognitive impairment.*

The purpose of the physical examination here is to find any clues to underlying medical or neurological disorders that may contribute to the cognitive impairment. For example, the examination may reveal clinical evidence of a treatable medical disorder such as hypothyroidism.

Laboratory studies that are usually included in the evaluation of suspected dementia include routine blood counts and chemistries that may indicate the presence of relevant systemic disease, as well as tests of thyroid function, vitamin levels (B-12 and folate) and a test for exposure to syphilis (because untreated latent syphilis may lead to dementia). Some clinicians include the apolipoprotein genotype test (see Chapter 4) in the diagnostic work-up.

The evaluation should also include a brain imaging test. Certain findings on such scans, specifically atrophy or hippocampal volume loss, may support a diagnosis of Alzheimer's disease; however, there are no specific findings indicative of Alzheimer's disease that can be shown on any imaging procedure. The primary purpose of including a brain scan in the evaluation is to look for evidence of an alternative diagnosis, such as vascular disease or normal pressure hydrocephalus (NPH, see below).

The most common methods of imaging the brain are the computerized tomography (CT) scan and the Magnetic Resonance Imaging (MRI) scan

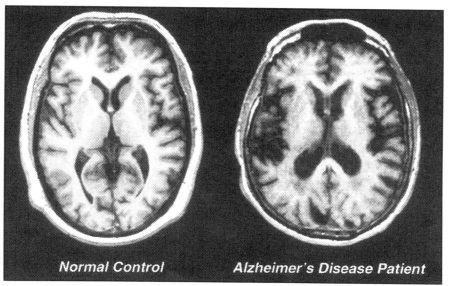

Figure 1.4 *Demonstrates an MRI scan of an individual with Alzheimer's disease (showing atrophy) compared with a normal control.*

ALZHEIMER'S DISEASE

(Figure 1.4). For the purpose of evaluating dementia, intravenous contrast (sometimes used to enhance the diagnostic resolution of CT scans) is usually not necessary, so there is virtually no discomfort or risk associated with these tests.

Both of these techniques provide images of brain structures. Newer techniques provide functional images of the brain. For example, Positron Emission Tomography (PET) scans provide images of cellular activity in various regions of the brain. Figure 1.5 compares a PET scan of an Alzheimer's patient to an individual without a memory disorder. The Alzheimer's image shows decreased cell functioning in the temporal and parietal lobes of the brain; these areas are involved in cognitive functioning.

While the history is the most important source of information regarding cognitive function, the evaluation of possible Alzheimer's disease also includes tests of cognitive ability. These tests range from brief screening tests done during the initial interview, to more in depth evaluations that may require multiple visits to a neuropsychologist.

The most commonly used cognitive screening test is the Folstein Mini-Mental State Examination, or MMSE. The MMSE consists of a series of questions that can be completed in a few minutes, and tests the patient's

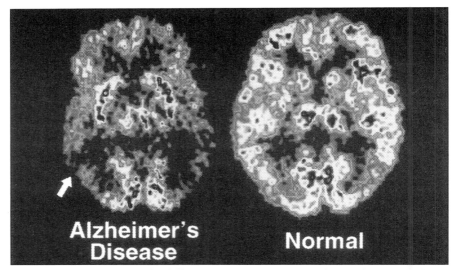

Figure 1.5 *Demonstrates the difference between PET scan of an individual with Alzheimer's disease and a normal brain. The marked region (with arrow) demonstrates decreased metabolism of the neuronal cells in the temporal and parietal lobes in the Alzheimer's brain.*

orientation, attention, language, and calculational ability. The result is a score, ranging from 0 to 30. Most patients with mild Alzheimer's disease score below 30; patients with severe dementia may score 0. However, while the MMSE is quite useful to clinicians, it has important limitations. Patients with mild Alzheimer's disease who are highly educated may get perfect scores on the MMSE, while patients with minimal education or who are not questioned in their primary language may get a low score in the absence of dementia.

What is the "eyedrop test" for Alzheimer's disease?

A recent study by a group of investigators at Harvard Medical School described a test using a commonly available eyedrop to distinguish patients with Alzheimer's disease from others. The eyedrop contains an anticholinergic medication (that is, a drug that blocks the effect of the chemical acetylcholine) that causes the pupil of the eye to dilate. Patients with Alzheimer's disease are generally abnormally sensitive to anticholinergic medications because the disease process itself depletes the brain of acetylcholine (acetylcholine is the most important chemical mediator of memory; see below). The investigators found that patients with Alzheimer's disease had more pupillary dilatation than did others in the study, suggesting that response to the eyedrop may be useful in establishing the diagnosis of Alzheimer's disease.

This study received a great deal of attention, because there is certainly a need for better diagnostic tools, and the eyedrop test is quick and easy to perform. However, before any proposed diagnostic test is accepted and incorporated into clinical practice, its utility must be confirmed by multiple studies in different settings. Follow-up studies of the eye-drop test have not confirmed its accuracy in distinguishing Alzheimer's disease from other dementing illnesses. Indeed, this experience is fairly typical: reports of new advances in the diagnosis or treatment of this disease receive a great deal of publicity, raising expectations which may well be dashed by follow-up studies.

Other screening tests for Alzheimer's disease that have been widely reported in the media are in fact cognitive tests that detect early deficits before the criteria for the diagnosis of dementia (see above) have been satisfied. In other words, cognitive tests can reveal mild impairments caused by a brain disease such as Alzheimer's disease in its early stages;

CAUSES OF DEMENTIA

◆ Alzheimer's disease   ◆ Vascular dementia

◆ Frontal lobe dementia   ◆ Parkinson's disease

◆ Normal pressure hydrocephalus ◆ Hypothyroidism

◆ B-12 deficiency   ◆ Neurosyphilis

◆ Major depression   ◆ Alcoholism

Figure 1.6 *Lists the major diagnostic considerations when evaluating an individual with dementia. Although there are over sixty causes of dementia, the illnesses listed above are the major illnesses underlying the development of dementia.*

but there is significant diagnostic inaccuracy in such screening procedures. They are, however, of value for following the clinical course of individuals with mild cognitive impairment.

What is the differential diagnosis of Alzheimer's disease?"

As discussed above, the first step in the diagnostic process is the determination of whether the subject meets the criteria for dementia. If dementia is present, the next step is the investigation of the cause or causes of the dementia. Figure 1.6 lists the most common causes of dementia that a clinician considers when evaluating a patient with cognitive impairment.

In elderly people, the most common cause of dementia is Alzheimer's disease. But this is a diagnosis of exclusion: there is no test (short of examination of brain tissue) that can establish the presence of Alzheimer's disease, so the diagnosis is made by excluding other possible causes.

The most important alternative explanation for dementia is vascular disease. Vascular dementia, also called multi-infarct dementia, occurs when there is loss of brain tissue resulting from occlusion of blood vessels (i.e. stroke, cerebral infarction) to an extent sufficient to cause global cognitive impairment. A single stroke will usually not cause dementia; there must be multiple strokes affecting both sides of the brain.

There is debate as to whether micro-infarctions not visible as discrete lesions on brain scans can cause dementia. Binswanger's Disease is a term sometimes applied to patients with dementia and multiple tiny infarcts.

With currently used clinical tools, it is not possible to distinguish Binswanger's disease from Alzheimer's disease. In the absence of multiple definite infarctions on CT or MRI, a diagnosis of Alzheimer's disease is generally appropriate.

Clinical history provides the only clues to the diagnosis of alcoholic dementia. A history of heavy chronic alcohol use in a patient with dementia suggests this diagnosis, particularly when the dementia does not progress after cessation of alcohol use.

What is the relationship between Frontal Lobe Dementia (FLD) and Alzheimer's disease?

There is a form of dementia, much less common than Alzheimer's disease, which involves primarily the frontal and temporal lobes of the brain with sparing of the parietal lobes. Pathologically, this condition is distinct from Alzheimer's disease: plaques and tangles are not found to the extent necessary to establish a diagnosis of Alzheimer's disease. A minority of these patients have distinct pathologic changes associated with Pick's Disease; most have no specific findings. The terms Frontal Lobe Dementia, Frontal-Temporal Dementia and Pick's Disease overlap, and are sometimes used interchangeably.

Clinically, there is some difference between FLD and Alzheimer's disease. In FLD, personality changes, disinhibition, and impaired judgment are generally more prominent early in the course of the illness than memory impairment and disorientation.

However, it is usually not possible to reliably distinguish between FLD and Alzheimer's disease on clinical grounds. Most patients ultimately found to have FLD on the basis of autopsy findings have been clinically diagnosed as Alzheimer's disease. Relatively new scanning techniques such as Proton Emission Tomography (or PET, an expensive procedure not widely available; see Figure 1.5) can be useful in distinguishing Alzheimer's disease from FLD.

It may not be critically important to attempt to distinguish Alzheimer's disease from FLD. There is no information available to suggest the response to any treatment intervention differs in the two diseases.

ALZHEIMER'S DISEASE

What is the relationship between Parkinson's disease and Alzheimer's disease?

Lewy Bodies are the pathologic findings in the brain that are characteristic of Parkinson's disease, a neurodegenerative disorder in which control of movement is the predominant clinical problem. In Parkinson's disease, Lewy Bodies in the basal ganglia, deep structures of the brain, result in what are termed "extra-pyramidal" symptoms (meaning symptoms caused by disease outside of the pyramidal tracts, the main motor pathways): bradykinesia or slowing of movements, rigidity, shuffling gait and tremor. In typical Parkinson's disease, cognitive impairment occurs only late in the illness.

However, there is considerable overlap between Alzheimer's disease and Parkinson's disease, both clinically and pathologically. It is not uncommon for extrapyramidal symptoms to occur in Alzheimer's disease, even in the absence of exposure to neuroleptic drugs (note that extrapyramidal symptoms are the most limiting side effects of neuroleptic drugs such as haloperidol, often prescribed to control behavioral symptoms in Alzheimer's disease; see Chapter 10). And the risk of dementia in patients with Parkinson's disease is double that of the general community population.

Neurotransmitters (discussed further in Chapter 4) are the chemicals that allow communication between connecting brain cells (neurons). Neurologic function depends not only on the absolute amounts of neurotransmitters, but also on the balance between neurotransmitters. Thus, extrapyramidal symptoms occur because of an imbalance between acetylcholine and dopamine. Such symptoms can be ameliorated not only by augmentation of dopaminergic neurotransmission, but also by blocking cholinergic neurotransmission; either intervention improves the balance between these classes of chemicals. Unfortunately, administering anticholinergic drugs to treat extrapyramidal symptoms often results in worsening of cognitive function, particularly when, as in patients with Alzheimer's disease, there is a pre-existing cholinergic deficit. For this reason, it is always preferable to treat extrapyramidal side effects of neuroleptic medication in Alzheimer's disease patients by reducing or eliminating the neuroleptic drug. If psychotic symptoms necessitate the use of antipsychotic medication, substitution of a lower potency neuroleptic, or an atypical neuroleptic such as risperidone or clozapine may improve the Parkinsonism.

When extrapyramidal symptoms are present early in Alzheimer's disease, or when Alzheimer's disease patients seem particularly prone to extrapyramidal side-effects of neuroleptic drugs (see below), Lewy Bodies may be found in the brain in addition to the usual plaques and tangles of Alzheimer's disease. This situation has been termed the Lewy-Body Variant of Alzheimer's disease.

On the other hand, when motor impairment is prominent early in the course of Alzheimer's disease, examination of the brain may indicate the widespread occurrence of Lewy Bodies beyond the basal ganglia. This has been called Diffuse Lewy Body Disease, or Dementia with Lewy Bodies.

In summary, there is a spectrum of neurodegenerative disease, from pure Alzheimer's disease, to the Lewy Body Variant of Alzheimer's disease and Diffuse Lewy Body Disease, to pure Parkinson's disease. Precise clinical differentiation of these conditions may not be possible. Clinicians must be aware of the potential for extrapyramidal symptoms and sensitivity to low dose neuroleptics in patients carrying the diagnosis of Alzheimer's disease, and of the appearance of cognitive dysfunction in Parkinson's disease patients, particularly when treated with anticholinergic drugs.

The term "Normal Pressure Hydrocephalus," or NPH, is often mentioned during the evaluation of a patient with cognitive decline. What is NPH?

The most important goal in the diagnostic evaluation of a patient with dementia is to determine whether any reversible cause or contributing factor is present. An example of a reversible type of dementia that appears similar to Alzheimer's disease is normal pressure hydrocephalus, or NPH. In this condition, there is an abnormal accumulation of cerebrospinal fluid (the fluid surrounding the brain and spinal cord) because of an impairment of resorption of the fluid. The build-up of fluid causes cognitive impairment, as well as, in most cases, ataxia (unsteady gait) and urinary incontinence. Each of these features can also be present in Alzheimer's disease, so it may be difficult to distinguish these two types of dementia solely by history and examination.

The CT or MRI scan is usually helpful in distinguishing NPH from Alzheimer's disease. In NPH, the accumulation of cerebrospinal fluid can be seen as an enlargement of the ventricles, cavities within the brain. In

Alzheimer's disease, the ventricles may also be enlarged (as a result of brain atrophy), but the sulci, grooves on the outer surface of the brain, are also enlarged, a finding not present in NPH.

NPH is a treatable disorder. In approximately 50% of cases, the cognitive impairment as well as the other manifestations of the disease improve following the surgival placement of a shunt to draint the cerebrospinal fluid. When the disgnosis of NPH is under consideration, neurologists may perform a series of spinal taps to remove cerebrospinal fluid. Clinical improvement after the spinal taps supports the diagnosis of NPH, and suggests that there may be sustained improvement after placement of a shunt.

Is accurate diagnosis of dementia possible? Is it important?

As discussed above, it is usually not possible to make a definitive diagnosis of Alzheimer's disease without examination of brain tissue. But in most cases, clinicians do not recommend brain biopsy. If treatable causes of dementia can be excluded with reasonable confidence, the information gained by brain biopsy does not justify the risks and discomforts associated with this procedure. In most cases in which a patient who had been diagnosed with Alzheimer's disease is found at autopsy to have another type of dementia, the correct diagnosis turns out to be a neurodegenerative (e.g. frontal lobe dementia, Lewy body disease) or vascular dementia, conditions without specific effective therapy. In these instances, an accurate antemortem diagnosis may not have substantially influenced the management.

Many families request post-mortem examination of the brain to definitively establish the cause of dementia. In addition to satisfying the natural desire to know the exact cause of disease, the information may be useful in considering risk of dementia to other family members. Post-mortem examination of brain tissue is a critically important component of Alzheimer's disease research programs.

What kind of physician diagnoses Alzheimer's disease?

A diagnosis of probable Alzheimer's disease can be made by a neurologist, psychiatrist, internist, geriatric specialist or family practitioner. The specialty of the clinician is less important than experience in the evaluation of dementia. Because Alzheimer's disease is so prevalent, many types of physicians have experience in making this diagnosis.

Unfortunately, it is quite common for patients and families to be dissatisfied with the interaction with the physician making the diagnosis. Many questions arise concerning the implications of the diagnosis and treatments available; a substantial amount of time must be allotted to discuss these issues. But changes in the health care system make it increasingly difficult for physicians to set aside enough time for such family discussions. Hearing the diagnosis of Alzheimer's disease is always associated with anxiety and discomfort; unanswered questions aggravate the situation with anger and resentment.

When a patient or family feels that they can benefit from more discussion regarding the symptoms or diagnosis, there are several options. A call to the Alzheimer's Association is often the best next step. Local chapters of the Alzheimer's Association are excellent sources of information about local counseling and support services, diagnostic centers, medical specialists and research programs.

If there is concern that the diagnostic evaluation has not been sufficiently thorough, or that other medical issues have not been resolved, a second opinion is worthwhile. Medical records including the results of all tests done during the dementia work-up should be brought to an appointment with an Alzheimer's Disease Center or a physician experienced in these issues.

What should a physician tell the patient with Alzheimer's disease?

It is always a difficult task for a physician to give a patient a diagnosis associated with fear and trepidation. In decades past, many physicians shielded their patients from "bad news" such as a diagnosis of cancer, to minimize suffering; medical decisions would be made by the physician, sometimes in consultation with family members. Now the accepted practice is to disclose all information to patients, and to share all medical decision-making with patients and their families.

Discussing the diagnosis of Alzheimer's disease is particularly challenging for several reasons. To many people, the diagnosis carries profoundly negative connotations, signifying senility, loss of control, total dependence.

ALZHEIMER'S DISEASE

The diagnosis can almost never be made definitively, so the discussion is further complicated by the uncertainty of "probable Alzheimer's disease." Finally, the affected individual often denies the existence of any problem, and may not have the capacity to understand or retain the relevant information.

Most physicians nonetheless adhere to the principle that all patients have a right to be fully informed of their condition and prognosis. When a physician arrives at the diagnosis of probable Alzheimer's disease, the conclusions and plans are discussed with the patient and family. It is obviously important that the physician address the patient, never referring to him/her in the third person. The discussion typically focuses on "memory loss," or "memory disorder;" use of the term "dementia" may be unnecessarily cruel. The physician may discuss the common occurrence of memory impairments with aging, and review the results of testing that failed to establish a definitive diagnosis. If the patient seems to be capable of understanding and receptive to the information, the physician will then explain that when no other cause for memory loss is uncovered, probable Alzheimer's disease is the diagnosis of exclusion. Particularly when the disease is in its early stages, some patients are grateful to participate in open, honest discussion of their condition, and may even express relief that they "are not crazy." After adequate discussion of the diagnosis, the patient and the family can consider appropriate care plans, safety measures and treatment options.

CHAPTER 2

EPIDEMIOLOGY

How common is Alzheimer's disease?

When discussing the rate of occurrence of a disease, epidemiologists distinguish between incidence (the rate at which new cases of a disease are diagnosed) and prevalence (the total number of cases of a disease, whether newly diagnosed or established, within a group).

Epidemiologic estimates for Alzheimer's disease vary a great deal from one study to another. This variability results in part from different methods used to define cases. There are many persons in the community who meet the clinical criteria for the diagnosis of probable Alzheimer's disease, but do not carry the diagnosis (the patient and/or family may not be aware of the extent of the cognitive impairment, or may have chosen not to seek medical evaluation). Incidence and prevalence figures will depend greatly on the measures taken to uncover cases of the disease.

Both the incidence and prevalence of Alzheimer's disease increase dramatically with age. The annual incidence rate rises from less than .5% among individuals in their sixties, to 3-6% by the late eighties. The prevalence of dementia (most people with dementia in fact have Alzheimer's disease) rises from about 1% among people in their early sixties, to between 25 and 50% among people in their late eighties. Most studies suggest that the prevalence of Alzheimer's disease doubles with every five years of age between 65 and 85, but this relationship does not hold for the very elderly (or every person over 100 would be demented, which is certainly not the case).

Why is the prevalence increasing?

Because the population of the U.S. and other developed countries is aging, any disease associated with aging is becoming more common. At present, there are an estimated 5 million cases of Alzheimer's disease in the U.S and it is expected that by the year 2040, there will be 7-10 million cases. While the figures are very rough estimates, the trend is unarguable. The

ALZHEIMER'S DISEASE

rising prevalence of Alzheimer's disease has vast implications for health care and economic planning, and should be an impetus to allocation of more funds to research.

CHAPTER 3

BRAIN FUNCTION AND ALZHEIMER'S DISEASE

What does the brain of the Alzheimer's patient look like?

At a post-mortem examination, the brain of a patient with Alzheimer's disease may or may not look grossly different from that of a person of similar age without the illness (see Figure 3.1). When it does appear different, it may look somewhat smaller, or atrophic, with widened spaces (called sulci) between ridges of brain tissue (called gyri). However, the classical changes in the Alzheimer's brain are seen under the microscope (See Figure 3.2). These abnormalities are called amyloid plaques and neurofibrillary tangles. Amyloid plaques are clumps of material deposited in the substance of the brain between nerve cells; the dense, insoluble material that constitutes these deposits is called amyloid.

For uncertain reasons, amyloid plaques are not evenly distributed throughout the brain. They occur primarily in those brain regions associated with cognitive function, particularly the temporal and parietal regions of the brain, with some extension into frontal areas. Rarely are there large numbers of plaques in other brain regions, such as the occipital lobe (involved in vision) and the cerebellum (balance and coordination).

Neurofibrillary tangles are clumps of material that form within nerve cells. Tangles are composed of proteins that are normally components of the backbone, or cytoskeleton, of the cell. The most important component of neurofibrillary tangles is tau, a protein that seems to be involved in the transport of materials within the cell. Compared with tau protein in normal cells, the tau in neurofibrillary tangles is chemically altered in a manner called hyperphosphorylation.

There are also more subtle abnormalities in the Alzheimer's brain. For example, there are changes that indicate an inflammatory response. Activated microglial cells, brain cells involved in inflammation, are found near amyloid plaques. Inflammatory proteins also accumulate in and around plaques.

ALZHEIMER'S DISEASE

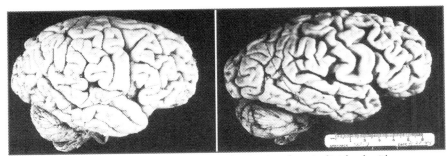

Figure 3.1 *This shows a normal brain and a brain of an individual with Alzheimer's disease. The Alzheimer's brain has widened sulci.*

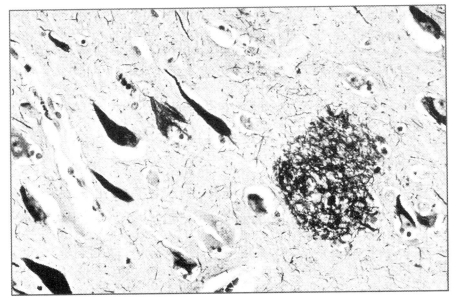

Figure 3.2 *This is a section of an Alzheimer's brain with the characteristic amyloid plaques and neurofibrillary tangles.*

It is worth noting that many healthy elderly people without Alzheimer's disease can have a relatively large number of plaques late in life. These individuals rarely have tangles as well. Though there is much speculation, it is not known why plaques sometimes cause the manifestations of Alzheimer's disease, while in some individuals they cause no apparent symptoms.

What are neurotransmitters, and how are they involved in Alzheimer's disease?

Neurotransmitters are the chemicals that allow communication between nerve cells. These chemicals are released by one nerve, and travel the short distance to stimulate a neighboring nerve cell. A deficiency of a neurotransmitter interferes with nerve cell communication, resulting in brain dysfunction.

While amyloid plaques and neurofibrillary tangles are the characteristic changes in brain tissue in Alzheimer's disease, it is the deficiency of neurotransmitters that develops as a result of the plaques and tangles that is probably the immediate cause of the clinical manifestations of the disease.

Many different chemicals act as neurotransmitters in the various regions of the brain. Despite the damage that exists in the Alzheimer's brain, quantities of many of these neurotransmitters are not markedly abnormal. Among those that are uniformly depleted are acetylcholine, corticotropin releasing factor, and somatostatin. Other neurotransmitters that may be deficient in the Alzheimer's brain include norepinephrine, serotonin, dopamine and glutamate.

Acetylcholine is the most important neurotransmitter in Alzheimer's disease. The deficiency of acetylcholine is the most dramatic and consistent, and it correlates most closely with the clinical manifestations of the illness. For many years, acetylcholine has been implicated as the primary neurotransmitter involved in memory and learning in experiments conducted in multiple species, including humans; thus the central role of acetylcholine depletion in Alzheimer's disease is not surprising. Indeed, the first drugs approved for the treatment of the cognitive symptoms of Alzheimer's disease, tacrine and donepezil, act by increasing brain levels of acetylcholine.

ALZHEIMER'S DISEASE

CHAPTER 4

WHAT IS KNOWN ABOUT THE CAUSE OF THE DISEASE?

In the past decade, our understanding of the processes in the brain that cause the decline in cognitive function characteristic of Alzheimer's disease has increased dramatically. But many crucial questions remain unanswered.

From the time of the early descriptions of cases of Alzheimer's disease, it has been known that the primary microscopic changes associated with the disease are the proteinaceous deposits called amyloid, along with abnormalities, called neurofibrillary tangles, that develop within brain cells. Determining the nature of these abnormal findings has yielded important insights into the cause of Alzheimer's disease. Characteristics of amyloid and neurofibrillary tangles are listed in Figures 4.1 and 4.2, respectively.

What is amyloid?

Amyloid is a medical term used to describe a protein that has certain characteristics when examined microscopically. Specifically, an amyloid protein has "apple-green birefringence" when examined with a polarizing microscope after staining with a dye called Congo red. This appearance indicates that the protein has a structure called "beta-pleated sheet." A number of different proteins have a beta-pleated sheet structure; the microscopic "amyloid" appearance does not distinguish among these proteins. But all of these proteins share certain features, such as insolubility and resistance to degradation, which probably account for their ability to cause disease by accumulating in body tissues.

There are several conditions called "amyloidoses" in which amyloid proteins accumulate in tissues causing disease. Various amyloidoses are characterized by deposition of amyloid proteins in the kidneys, liver, heart or peripheral nerves, causing dysfunction of the affected organs. In Alzheimer's disease, amyloid protein is deposited in the brain tissue itself and in blood vessels within the brain; the result is brain dysfunction, or dementia. (Actually, this is a simplification. Amyloid accumulates in the brain, and brain cells are injured, but whether the former directly causes the latter is uncertain. Other abnormal processes within the brain, such as the accumulation of neurofibrillary tangles within neurons, may be crucially important).

Where does the amyloid protein come from?

In Alzheimer's disease, the specific amyloid protein has been named "beta-amyloid" or "amyloid beta-protein." The precise composition of this small protein, consisting of about 42 amino acids, is known. Beta-amyloid derives from a larger protein, aptly called the amyloid precursor protein (APP). APP is normally produced by a number of different types of cells in the body; the function of this protein is not completely understood. APP is normally situated partially within the outer membrane of cells. By metabolic pathways not fully understood, APP can be broken down into beta-amyloid, which in turn deposits in the brain; extensive deposition of beta-amyloid in the brain is associated with Alzheimer's disease.

Does deposition of amyloid protein in the brain cause dementia?

Many (but by no means all) researchers have concluded that deposition of amyloid protein in the brain is the key event leading to the development of Alzheimer's disease. One reason is simply that dying brain cells can be found surrounding the amyloid deposits in regions of the brain important to memory and other cognitive functions. But another compelling clue that amyloid deposition is key was uncovered by the careful study of families with an autosomal dominant form of Alzheimer's disease. Such kindreds account for a very small proportion of all cases of Alzheimer's disease, but for neuroscientists they are critically important to understanding the disease.

If a disease is transmitted from one generation to the next in an autosomal dominant manner, meaning that the odds that a child of an affected parent will also have the disease is 50%, it can be concluded that the disease is caused by the product of a single gene. Discovering the product of that gene should reveal the cause of the disease. For a few families with autosomal dominant inheritance of Alzheimer's disease, the defective gene was identified as the gene for the amyloid precursor protein. In other words, in a small number of families, carrying a gene which codes for an abnormal form of APP causes Alzheimer's disease. Though the vast majority of patients with Alzheimer's disease have a normal APP gene, the fact that an abnormal APP gene can cause Alzheimer's disease suggests that APP and its products (i.e. beta-amyloid protein) play a central role in the disease.

A second important observation that supports the notion that APP metabolism is key to the development of Alzheimer's disease is the occurrence of Alzheimer's disease in most individuals with Down syndrome who survive beyond age 50 (autopsy studies have shown that essentially all older individuals with Down syndrome have plaques and tangles characteristic of Alzheimer's disease; most show the clinical features of dementia in their fifties). Down syndrome is caused by trisomy 21, the presence of an extra chromosome 21. The APP gene is located on chromosome 21, so Down's patients have an extra copy of the APP gene. It seems reasonable to conclude that an extra "dose" of the APP gene results in the early development of Alzheimer's disease in these patients.

How might the same disease occur in patients with an abnormal or extra APP gene and those with a normal APP gene? Perhaps APP is normally broken down mainly into harmless fragments. The abnormal APP that is present in a few families might resist the normal degradation pathway, but rather favor a secondary pathway that produces harmful amyloid fragments. As a result of the extra copy of the APP gene, individuals with Down syndrome may produce too much APP, overwhelming the normal degradation pathway, leading to the accumulation of the harmful fragments. In the majority of Alzheimer's disease patients with normal APP, some other abnormality might block the normal safe pathway and favor the generation of amyloid fragments.

How can the deposition of amyloid be prevented?

If the breakdown of APP into amyloid fragments that deposit in brain tissue is a central event in the development of Alzheimer's disease, then several treatment strategies become evident. First, drugs which suppress the production by cells of APP might slow the process of amyloid deposition. Second, drugs which alter the degradation of APP into amyloid fragments, by favoring the production of safe "non-amyloidogenic" products, should also be beneficial. And finally, drugs which inhibit the deposition of amyloid fragments into plaques, or accelerate the resorption of amyloid that

A LZHEIMER'S DISEASE

Where do free radicals fit into this scenario?

Free radicals (also called reactive oxygen species) such as superoxide and hydroxyl radicals are molecules that have unpaired electrons and therefore react violently with other molecules, disrupting, for example, critical cell membrane constituents. Damaging free radical reactions may require the presence of metal ions, such as iron. Free radicals are generated by normal metabolic processes, and are a necessary component of the body's defense against infection. To minimize damage to tissues, the body has protective mechanisms that limit the activity of free radicals.

Some gerontologists and neuroscientists believe that tissue damage from free radicals contributes to aging in general and Alzheimer's disease in particular. There is evidence of free radical damage in the brain in Alzheimer's disease, though it remains unclear whether free radicals contribute to the disease in an important way. Some have advocated that all people take antioxidant vitamins, particularly vitamins C and E, to protect against damage from free radicals. But there is no evidence to support this recommendation, and it should be remembered that all medications including vitamins can cause adverse effects.

There are ongoing clinical trials examining the effects of antioxidants with regard to Alzheimer's disease. One carefully controlled trial did show evidence that high dose vitamin E treatment (1000 IU twice daily) taken by patients in the moderate stage of Alzheimer's disease may slow the clinical progression of the disease. There is no conclusive evidence at this time that vitamin E (or any other treatment) reduces the risk of developing Alzheimer's disease.

What is the role of inflammation in Alzheimer's disease?

The body has evolved a complex set of mechanisms, collectively termed the inflammatory response, to combat infection. In some diseases (rheumatoid arthritis and lupus erythematosus are examples), inflammatory mechanisms are directed not against invading organisms, but rather against the body's own tissues. In these diseases, anti-inflammatory medications can ameliorate symptoms and limit tissue damage.

During the past ten years, scientists have discovered that inflammatory has already been laid down, might improve the course of the disease. Each of these strategies is currently being explored in research programs.

What are neurofibrillary tangles?

The second microscopic abnormality present in the brain in Alzheimer's disease is the neurofibrillary tangle. This term describes the appearance within neurons of dense cytoskeletal (structural) proteins. Neurofibrillary tangles are not unique to Alzheimer's disease, and are not uniformly present in elderly patients with Alzheimer's disease. Nonetheless, they seem to mark neuronal cell injury, and some studies suggest that these structures correlate closely with the clinical manifestations of the disease.

Much attention has focused on one particular protein component of neurofibrillary tangle, called tau protein. The tau protein found within tangles in Alzheimer's disease differs from tau protein in normal brain. Tau protein in Alzheimer's disease brain has been chemically modified; specifically, it is phosphorylated. Some neuroscientists speculate that phosphorylation of tau and other proteins may be an important process leading to cellular dysfunction in Alzheimer's disease. Blocking the phosphorylation of tau may represent a therapeutic strategy.

Which is more important: amyloid plaques or neurofibrillary tangles?

There is active debate among researchers concerning the relative importance of plaques and tangles to the development of Alzheimer's disease. Some studies indicate that neurofibrillary tangles, though they are not specific to Alzheimer's disease, correlate more closely than plaques with clinical features of the disease. On the other hand, a mutation in the APP gene is definitely linked to familial Alzheimer's disease, and it seems likely that the reason Alzheimer's disease develops prematurely in patients with Down syndrome is that they carry an extra copy of the APP gene.

The direct cause of cognitive decline is presumably the loss of neurons and synapses, the connections between neurons, along with deficiencies of neurotransmitters. Perhaps increased production of amyloid protein is an early, critical step, while the tangles mark the death of neurons from exposure to amyloid protein or other toxic compounds, such as free radicals and inflammatory proteins.

mechanisms are active in the Alzheimer's disease brain. It is possible (but not proven) that inflammation contributes to the loss of brain function, and that anti-inflammatory medication may be helpful. Surveys by a number of investigators suggest that use of anti-inflammatory drugs may be associated with a lower risk of Alzheimer's disease, but such surveys are never conclusive. As discussed further in the next chapter, it is essential to conduct controlled clinical trials to determine whether anti-inflammatory drugs are useful in Alzheimer's disease. Such trials are now in progress.

CHARACTERISTICS OF AMYLOID PROTEIN

◆ Almyloid is a 42 amino acid protein with a beta pleated sheet structure

◆ Amyloid derives from a larger protein, amyloid precursor protein (APP)

◆ Increased deposition of amyloid in the brain is characterisitc of Alzheimer's disease

◆ Amyloid deposition may be a critical step in the development of Alzheimer's disease

---

Figure 4.1 *Lists essential characteristics of amyloid protein and its relationship to Alzheimer's disease.*

CHARACTERISTICS OF NEUROFIBRILLARY TANGLES

◆ Neurofibrillary tangles are proteins found in neuronal cells in Alzheimer's disease

◆ Neurofibrillary tangles are markers of neuronal cell injury

◆ Phosphorylated tau protein is a prominent features of neurofibrillary tangles

◆ Formation of neurofibrillary tangles may be a critical step in the development of Alzheimer's disease

---

Figure 4.2 *Lists essential characteristics of neurofibrillary tangles and their relationship to Alzheimer's disease.*

CHAPTER 5

ARE THERE ANY RISK FACTORS FOR ALZHEIMER'S DISEASE?

A number of factors appear to increase the likelihood that an individual will eventually develop Alzheimer's disease (see Figure 5.1). Most of these factors appear to be beyond an individual's control.

The most compelling risk factor for Alzheimer's disease is age. The striking relationship between an individual's age and the likelihood of developing Alzheimer's disease is one of the most obvious features of this disorder. Alzheimer's disease is relatively uncommon in individuals between ages 65-69; its incidence is more than ten-fold greater in people over the age of 80.

Other than age, are there important risk factors for Alzheimer's disease?

A family history of Alzheimer's disease, and the presence of one specific form of the gene for a substance called apolipoprotein E, are also definite risk factors for Alzheimer's disease.

How do genes influence a person's risk for Alzheimer's disease?

The impact of genetics on Alzheimer's disease is quite complex. It is clear that there are some families that have a very strong genetic component to the disease. For example, there are a few kindreds (extended families) with

---

RISK FACTORS FOR ALZHEIMER'S DISEASE

◆ Increasing age   ◆ Inheritence of certain genes

◆ Family history of dementia   ◆ Less eduction

Figure 5.1 *Lists several risk factors that have been implicated in the development of Alzheimer's disease. While no one factor can predict the development of the illness, this information can be clincially meaningful and important for research efforts.*

autosomal dominant transmission. This means that a person in such a family who has a parent with Alzheimer's disease would have a 50% chance of also having the disease. These pedigrees are extremely rare, and are characterized by a very early age of onset of Alzheimer's disease, sometimes below the age of 50. However, such families have been quite informative in elucidating some of the molecular underpinnings of Alzheimer's disease. For example, it has been determined in some of these kindreds that mutations in the amyloid precursor protein gene are responsible for the very high genetic prevalence of Alzheimer's disease in these families. This finding has convinced many researchers that the key to the cause of Alzheimer's disease lies in an understanding of the metabolic pathways of the amyloid precursor protein (see also Chapter 3).

What is meant by sporadic versus familial Alzheimer's disease?

A "sporadic" case of a disease with a genetic basis is a case that occurs in a family with no other known cases of the disease. When Alzheimer's disease occurs in a family with no family history of Alzheimer's disease, it is clearly "sporadic". Conversely, when Alzheimer's disease occurs in a family in which there has been a history of Alzheimer's disease, it may loosely be considered "familial". However, because Alzheimer's disease is most common in people over the age of 80, while the average person does not survive beyond the age of 80, many Alzheimer's disease patients classified as sporadic may actually have a familial form of the disease; if other close family members had lived long enough, they might have developed the disease. Because of the high prevalence of Alzheimer's disease among elderly people, most individuals with elderly family members will have a "positive family history" of Alzheimer's disease.

A more restrictive and perhaps more practical use of the term familial Alzheimer's disease includes only families in which the disease is inherited in a autosomal dominant manner. Many experts consider all cases not fitting this restrictive definition of familial Alzheimer's disease to have sporadic disease. With this usage of the term, about 95% of cases of Alzheimer's disease are sporadic.

If I have a brother, sister, mother, or father with Alzheimer's disease, how is my risk of the disease affected?

As with any disease that has some genetic component, a family history of

Alzheimer's disease generally increases one's likelihood of developing the disease. However, the relationship between a family history and the likelihood of Alzheimer's disease is affected by the age of onset of the family member who suffered from Alzheimer's disease; a relatively young age of onset may indicate a stronger genetic component.

Have any specific genes been linked to Alzheimer's disease?

Mutations on chromosome 21, specifically in the amyloid precursor protein (APP) gene, have been associated with familial Alzheimer's disease in a very few families. A number of distinct mutations in this gene have been associated with the disease. While these mutations account for only a tiny fraction of cases, their existence is an important clue that APP plays a central role in the development of the disease. This notion is further supported by the fact that Alzheimer's disease develops at a young age in subjects with Down's syndrome, as discussed above; in this genetic disorder, there is an extra copy of chromosome 21, and therefore an extra copy of the APP gene.

More recently, genes on chromosomes 1 and 14 have been linked to familial Alzheimer's disease. The function of the proteins, called presenilins, coded by these genes is not yet understood, but they may play a role in the metabolism of APP. The discovery of the link between Alzheimer's disease and these two genes has generated enormous excitement; further research in this area is likely to lead to major insights into the cause of Alzheimer's disease.

Another recent breakthrough has been the discovery that specific forms (alleles) of the gene for a protein called apolipoprotein E that an individual carries are related to the risk of developing sporadic Alzheimer's disease. The gene for apolipoprotein E is located on chromosome 19.

How strong a risk factor for Alzheimer's disease is apolipoprotein E genotype?

There are a three different alleles for apolipoprotein E, labeled E2, E3, and E4 (or sometimes epsilon 2,3 and 4). It is clear that having the apolipoprotein E4 allele on each of the two copies of chromosome 19 (i.e., being homozygous for E4) greatly increases one's risk for Alzheimer's disease. Having only one apolipoprotein E4 allele also increases the

ALZHEIMER'S DISEASE

likelihood of developing Alzheimer's disease. Thus, while 25-30% of the general population carries the E4 allele, half or more of patients with Alzheimer's disease carry E4. There is suggestive but preliminary evidence that the presence of the E2 allele might actually decrease one's risk of Alzheimer's disease.

What is apolipoprotein E, and why should it affect one's risk for Alzheimer's disease?

Apolipoproteins are involved in the transport and metabolism of lipids. They are important in the metabolism of cholesterol, and therefore have a significant role in the development of cardiovascular disease. The role of apolipoprotein E in the central nervous system is not entirely clear. However, it is known that lipid reorganization is necessary for the normal function of the nervous system, and that apolipoproteins may play an important role in reorganizing the lipid structure of nerve cell membranes. There is also evidence that apolipoprotein E is involved in the transport and disposition of amyloid fragments. Further, studies suggest that the E2, E3 and E4 forms of apolipoprotein differ in ability to transport amyloid proteins, and thus influence either the deposition of amyloid, or the processing of the amyloid precursor protein. Whatever the mechanism, it is clear that the presence of apolipoprotein E4 is a strong risk factor. This discovery is an essential lead in helping to understand Alzheimer's disease, and ultimately developing an effective treatment.

Should members of our family be tested for apolipoprotein E genotype?

While the link between apolipoprotein E and Alzheimer's disease is an important discovery, determination of apolipoprotein E genotype is not sufficiently sensitive or specific to be useful by itself as a diagnostic test for Alzheimer's disease. In addition, it is not recommended as a test to predict later development of the disease. Many subjects who carry the apolipoprotein E4 allele will never develop the disease, and some who do not have this risk factor will develop Alzheimer's disease. Because at the present time there is no intervention proven to delay the occurrence of Alzheimer's disease, quantifying one's risk using apolipoprotein E genotype is not particularly useful.

Since there is always some uncertainty to the clinical diagnosis of Alzheimer's disease, some experts have incorporated apolipoprotein genotype testing into the diagnostic evaluation. The presence of the apolipoprotein E4 allele increases the likelihood that the cause of cognitive decline is in fact Alzheimer's disease. It has been estimated that apolipoprotein E genotyping improves the accuracy of diagnosis by about 5%.

Is aluminum a risk factor for Alzheimer's disease?

Aluminum has been found to be associated with the changes in brain tissue that occur in Alzheimer's disease. This has led to the suggestion that aluminum may in some way facilitate the development of Alzheimer's disease, but this notion has not been proven. Epidemiological studies have not yielded any clear evidence linking environmental exposure to aluminum with the disease.

Experts have concluded that there is no cause for concern about aluminum intake or the use of aluminum pots and pans in the home.

Is zinc a risk factor for Alzheimer's disease?

Evidence linking zinc to Alzheimer's disease is much more scant than that for aluminum. Some laboratory studies indicate that there may be important interactions between zinc and amyloid protein. However there is no clear evidence that environmental exposure to zinc, or the use of nutritional supplements containing zinc, is either beneficial or harmful with regard to Alzheimer's disease.

What is the relationship between Down syndrome and Alzheimer's disease?

As discussed in Chapter 4, Down syndrome is definitely a very strong risk factor for Alzheimer's disease. Individuals with Down syndromes have an extra copy of chromosome 21. The gene for the amyloid precursor protein (APP) resides on chromosome 21, so individuals with Down syndrome have an extra copy of this gene; they have 50% greater capacity than others to generate APP. Since APP is the source of beta-amyloid protein, the primary constituent of the amyloid plaques that deposit in the Alzheimer's disease brain, it is not surprising that individuals with Down syndrome are highly susceptible to Alzheimer's disease. Indeed, essentially all adults with Down syndrome over the age of thirty have brain amyloid deposits, and most develop the clinical manifestations of Alzheimer's disease in their forties or fifties. As noted in Chapter 4, the link between Down syndrome and Alzheimer's disease has strengthened the theory that amyloid deposits are a central etiologic feature of the illness.

Are there any factors that may decrease the risk for Alzheimer's disease?

There is fairly strong evidence that there is an inverse relationship between years of education and risk of Alzheimer's disease. Some have theorized that education increases "brain reserve", increasing resistence to the clinical manifestations of the disease. But the apparent protective effect of higher education may just be an artifact of the standard diagnostic procedures. Educated people generally obtain high scores on cognitive screening tests such as the Mini-Mental State Examination (MMSE); their scores typically remain in the normal range during the early stages of dementing illness. More challenging cognitive tests may reveal substantial decline, and support a diagnosis of Alzheimer's disease even in an individual with a perfect score on the MMSE. Similarly, the casual questioning and simple cognitive tasks that often yield evidence of dementia during a clinical interview may not reveal any deficit in a highly educated person in the early stage of Alzheimer's disease. The apparent protective effect of education may thus be explained by the greater difficulty involved in demonstrating mild cognitive deficits in persons with advanced education.

Is estrogen protective against Alzheimer's disease?

A number of epidemiologic surveys suggest that use of estrogen by post-menopausal women reduces the risk or slows the course of Alzheimer's disease. These studies are certainly not conclusive, however. Use of estrogen may be more common among women with higher education and better access to health care, and such women may have a lower rate of Alzheimer's disease; thus estrogen use may be a marker of reduced risk, rather than a drug that actually reduces risk. On the other hand, basic laboratory research has provided plausible mechanisms by which estrogen might be protective. There is a great deal of interest in this area, and controlled clinical trials are now underway to determine whether estrogen use offers benefits with regard to Alzheimer's disease. At this time, many experts do not consider these possible benefits of estrogen to be as important as the well-established benefits (such as protection against osteoporosis) and risks (effects on breast and uterine cancer, and thromboembolism). Decisions regarding estrogen use are often difficult, and must be made in consultation with a knowledgeable physician.

Does aspirin or ibuprofen protect against Alzheimer's disease?

Although few neuroscientists would suggest that Alzheimer's disease is totally a consequence of inflammation in the brain, there is undoubtedly an inflammatory brain reaction that occurs in the Alzheimer's patient, as mentioned in the preceding chapter. Most investigators believe that this inflammatory response is secondary to the primary abnormalities (amyloid plaques and degenerating neurons) characteristic of the Alzheimer's disease brain. Figure 5.2 reviews the evidence supporting the role of inflammation in Alzheimer's disease. However, whether the course of Alzheimer's disease may in some way be modulated (i.e. slowed) by the administration of anti-inflammatory drugs remains a critical question. A large number of epidemiological surveys suggest that the use of anti-inflammatory agents such as nonsteroidal anti-inflammatory drugs (e.g. ibuprofen), and perhaps even aspirin, might decrease the risk and/or progression rate of Alzheimer's disease. In fact, one pilot study with a small number of patients suggested an advantage to those Alzheimer's patients taking the anti-inflammatory drug

---

ROLE OF INFLAMMATION IN ALZHEIMER'S DISEASE

◆ Inflammatory molecules and cells accumulate around amyloid plaques in Alzheimer's disease

◆ In laboratory studies, these inflammatory mediators are toxic to brain cells

◆ The inflammatory response may be secondary to the primary lesion in Alzheimer's disease

◆ Whether anti-inflammatory agents are useful in the prevention or treatment of Alzheimer's disease is under study

---

Figure 5.2 *Summarizes the role of inflammation in Alzheimer's disease.*

indomethacin compared to a control group taking a placebo. These intriguing studies have led to the initiation of several large multicenter studies in the United States and in Europe of various anti-inflammatory drug regimens. As with estrogen, the evidence in support of a benefit of anti-inflammatory drugs is not yet strong enough to justify recommending their use.

It should be noted that while aspirin is an effective anti-inflammatory drug at high doses (12 to 20 tablets per day), at the low doses recommended for cardiovascular benefits, aspirin has no anti-inflammatory activity. It thus seems unlikely that one aspirin per day will be useful in the treatment or prevention of Alzheimer's disease.

The possibility of preventing or treating Alzheimer's disease with anti-inflammatory drugs is discussed further in Chapter 9.

Can antioxidants, and even the antioxidant vitamins, diminish the likelihood of Alzheimer's disease?

It was mentioned in the preceding chapter (and discussed further in Chapter 9) that free radicals, molecules with unpaired electrons, can be destructive to cells. With the hope of diminishing the consequences of free radical production, antioxidants have been suggested as a treatment to decrease the likelihood of developing Alzheimer's disease or to slow the disease course. One controlled study has demonstrated that use of high doses of vitamin E or the antioxidant medication selegeline may slow the clinical progression of Alzheimer's disease when administered to patients in the moderate stage of the disease. Another trial suggested that use of one formulation of ginkgo biloba, a supplement that may have antioxidant properties, slightly slows cognitive decline in Alzheimer's disease. Because vitamin E is a potent antioxidant that is widely available, relatively inexpensive, and has few side effects, many experts now recommend its use. The optimal dose and timing of treatment are not known; a high dose, 1000 IU twice daily, has been advocated because this dose was effective in the controlled trial. A large trial to determine whether vitamin E can delay or prevent the disease has now been started. As with all medications and supplements, prescription and over-the-counter, vitamin E does have risks. For example, vitamin E can cause bleeding problems in people taking anticoagulants.

CHAPTER 6

WHAT ARE THE CLINICAL MANIFESTATIONS OF ALZHEIMER'S DISEASE?

Deborah B. Marin and Jennifer Hoblyn

What are the symptoms of Alzheimer's disease?

Patients with Alzheimer's disease have difficulty with thinking (cognition), behavior patterns, and day-to-day functioning. Cognition includes memory, orientation, language, judgement and problem-solving. Behavior patterns encompass personality, mood, activity level, and perceptions of the environment. Day-to-day function refers to the ability to work, take care of personal needs and the home, and participate in the community. As the illness progresses, the affected individual experiences increasing challenges in each of these areas.

Alzheimer's disease is often divided into mild, moderate, and severe stages. Staging aids in understanding the typical signs and symptoms of the illness that are likely to aggregate with one another. Each stage that is described below can last a few years. Therefore, the changes that are described are gradual, and not apparent on a day-to-day basis. This chapter describes the clinical symptoms of Alzheimer's disease according to the stages in an effort to elucidate the course of the illness.

What changes in memory occur in Alzheimer's disease?

Memory problems must be present to support a diagnosis of Alzheimer's disease. Typically, memory is the first cognitive domain to be affected by the illness. The memory loss must represent a decline from the individual's usual memory ability; it differs from the static complaint of absent-mindedness that many normal individuals report. The memory loss is also distinguishable from the occasional minor memory impairment that may occur with normal aging. In Alzheimer's disease, this problem is consistent, occurs with difficulties in at least one other area of cognition, and is associated with decline in day-to-day functioning.

In mild Alzheimer's disease, the memory loss is usually restricted to recent events, while recollection of past events is spared. For example, the patient may forget details of recent social functions and conversations yet have excellent recall for events that occurred 20 years ago. This memory problem typically causes the Alzheimer's disease patient to repeatedly ask the same questions. The individual in the mild stage may recall some events very well, or recall portions of events. The memory problems occur because the brain's capacity to learn new information, like a telephone number, name, or location of an appointment, is impaired.

Memory impairment, like other cognitive and behavioral aspects of this disease, cannot be controlled by the patient. It is harmful, rather than helpful, for family or friends to blame the patient for these deficits. Family members often note that their relative with Alzheimer's disease may become excessively irritable when confronted with the memory loss.

The memory loss may affect the ability to perform daily activities such as shopping, cooking or keeping appointments. Recalling events with the patient, or offering names of friends in social situations, can be very helpful. Often, patients are not aware of the intensity of their memory problem. Therefore, a loved one who has concern about an individual's memory may have to initiate a consultation with the patient's primary physician. Figure 6.1 lists some typical signs of memory loss in mild Alzheimer's disease.

**TYPICAL SIGNS OF THE MEMORY LOSS
IN MILD ALZHEIMER'S DISEASE**

◆ Forgetfulness of recent events is greater than for remote events

◆ The same questions are asked repeatedly

◆ Learning new information is impaired

◆ The memory impairment is consistent

Figure 6.1 *Lists the signs of memory loss observed in mild Alzheimer's disease. As noted, the loss is primarily for recent events and is consistent.*

In the moderate stage of Alzheimer's disease, memory of recent events is more limited. At this point, the individual almost certainly does not recall recent conversations or activities. Typically, only highly learned material is retained (e.g., one's birthday or place of birth). The Alzheimer's disease patient may not always remember the names or identities of family members or long-time friends. This memory loss is often of great concern to people who are close to the patient. At this stage, reminiscing about enjoyable experiences may be very therapeutic for the patient. Such interactions provides an opportunity to focus on memories that are most likely to be intact. As in the mild stage of the illness, reminding the affected individual about their deficits is more psychologically stressful than beneficial.

In the severe stage of the illness, the Alzheimer's disease patient displays significant difficulty with long-term memory as well. The individual is likely to fail to recall any names of individuals whom he/she has known for years. On the other hand, a caring interaction (e.g. holding the patient's hands, singing, or soothing conversation) is often associated with a positive response by the patient.

How does Alzheimer's disease affect one's orientation?

The term orientation includes three "spheres": time (date, day of the week, month, year, season), place (place of residence, neighborhood), and person (knowledge of one's and others' identity). Loss of orientation usually progresses from the sphere of time, to place, and lastly to person. This sequence of loss of orientation is consistent with progression through the three stages of Alzheimer's disease.

In the mild stage, Alzheimer's disease patients may be completely oriented to the exact date and location, and to self. However, time relationships (i.e., when events exactly happen) may be slightly impaired. For example, a patient with mild Alzheimer's disease may get ready for an appointment hours or even days before the scheduled time. He or she may also repeatedly ask the time of an upcoming social event. Orientation in one's familiar surroundings is usually very good. Slight difficulty in unfamiliar surroundings may occur. As a consequence, the Alzheimer's disease patient may have difficulty navigating from one place to another outside of his/her own neighborhood.

In the moderate stage, the patient with Alzheimer's disease is often disoriented to time, often not knowing the date or year. The disorientation in time can be manifested as the belief that he/she is living in an earlier period of his/her life. Consequently, he/she may believe that deceased relatives are still alive or that his/her grown children are still youngsters. The disorientation to place may be evident in the patient's own home. The Alzheimer's disease patient may not recall where to place dishes or linens. This problem often leads to household objects being misplaced. The individual may repeatedly ask to "go home", even when in his/her own house. Redirecting the patient to another activity and calm reassurance are helpful responses from family and friends. Proper supervision aids the patient with activities in the home, and protects against getting lost. There are several effective and safe methods to protect the patient from wandering (see Chapter 7).

In the severe stage, the Alzheimer's disease patient gradually loses all spheres of orientation. He/she is unable to provide the correct date, and consistently needs help with orientation in the home. The patient may respond to his/her own name, but have difficulty repeating it. Recognition of family members is primarily nonverbal. At this stage, a consistent environment and daily routines are calming for the patient.

How is language affected in Alzheimer's disease?

As people age, they often complain that they have difficulty retrieving words, especially names. However, they subsequently recall the correct word, and this problem neither interferes with day-to-day functioning nor is significantly progressive. Upon casual encounter, the mild Alzheimer's disease patient may appear to have this type of mild word-finding difficulty. However, neuropsychological testing often identifies significant difficulties with naming objects, especially complex or infrequently used words.

In the moderate stage of the illness, word-finding difficulty is more apparent. The individual's speech is less spontaneous and complex. Since the amount of speech is diminished, the person may appear withdrawn. Word substitutions become more common; for example, the term "the thing that tells time" might be used for "watch". At times, the patient may be difficult to understand. Since commonly used phrases may not be affected, the Alzheimer's disease patient may rely heavily on these during conversations.

During the severe stage of Alzheimer's disease, the affected individual has difficulty producing complete sentences. Speech is often hard to understand, and not necessarily related to environmental events. The patient at this stage may best communicate in a non-verbal fashion. Alzheimer's disease patients may display a speech pattern characterized by echolalia (i.e., echoing what is heard) or palilalia (i.e. repeating sounds or words over and over).

How are problem solving and judgment affected in Alzheimer's disease?

Problem solving and judgement refer to the ability to appropriately handle the day-to-day challenges that occur at home, work, or in social situations. Impairments in these areas are observed in the mild stage of the illness if the individual is faced with complex tasks. For example, planning and preparing a dinner party, balancing the checkbook, or conducting financial transactions may be increasingly challenging. In contrast, performing simple household chores or routine shopping may be completely normal. The individual's ability to integrate new information, e.g. in the news or in their personal life, may be affected. Learning how to use a new household appliance may be unusually challenging. It is important that individuals in the mild stage make provisions regarding the handling of finances (see the chapter on Legal Planning): Patients in the mild stage of the disease are at risk of making bad business decisions, or inappropriately giving money away.

In the moderate stage, the Alzheimer's disease patient can no longer manage money. The patient is unable to make change or leave an appropriate tip in a restaurant. At this stage, the patient has more difficulty grasping novel situations, like news, movies, or social events. Performing simple household chores, e.g. making the bed, may be intact. However, using the microwave, remote control, or VCR may be very difficult.

In the moderate stage, the Alzheimer's patient is likely to have difficulty handling a household emergency or appropriately responding to a stranger at the door. He/she is at risk of forgetting to turn off the stove or running water. In order to avoid a possibly dangerous situation, the caregivers should arrange for comprehensive supervision of the patient.

In the severe stage of Alzheimer's disease, the capacity to solve problems is significantly impaired. Decisions regarding what to wear or eat need to be supervised. There is generally no pretense of independent problem solving at this stage.

ALZHEIMER'S DISEASE

What impact does Alzheimer's disease have on an individual's involvement in the community?

Community affairs refer to activities the individual performs outside of the home, either alone or with others. In the mild stage of the illness, the Alzheimer's disease patient may perform quite independently and meaningfully in his/her community. He/she may be able to do shopping in local stores and go to the local barber or hairdresser without much problem. The ability to participate in a meaningful manner in senior groups and volunteer organizations may also be largely preserved. Participation in card games or sports may be well maintained. Some supervision may be needed, but overall the individual maintains much of his/her functioning in the community.

As the disease progresses to the moderate stage, highly learned activities, like picking up the local paper, may be maintained. However, at this stage there should not be the expectation that the individual can function independently in the community. Shopping becomes problematic, with the Alzheimer's disease patient buying duplicate items while forgetting necessities. Senior center involvement may be more limited, since many activities in such settings lack the necessary supervision and are too complex. Some patients at this stage may continue to perform hobbies well.

Alzheimer's disease patients often do not initiate involvement in social situations. This avoidance can mimic the social withdrawal seen in depression. In contrast to a depressed patient, an Alzheimer's individual will relate how much they enjoy activities. At times, the individual may behave inappropriately in social situations: he/she may use crass words, or be overly disinhibited. Nonetheless, the patient usually appears well enough to be taken to social events.

In the severe stage of the illness, the Alzheimer's disease patient appears frail. He/she may be able to engage in social functions in a limited fashion. However, other community activities may be too demanding, even with supervision. The individual may do best with activities in the home.

What about driving?

Driving problems may occur even in the mild stage of Alzheimer's disease. Examples include impaired depth perception and speed control, difficulty navigating to familiar places, or slowed responses to lights and stop signs. It is not possible to accurately predict when a major problem, such as a serious accident, will occur. Even in mild Alzheimer's disease, the patient may become momentarily disoriented or may react incorrectly in dangerous situations. Thus, driving is not recommended for any patient with Alzheimer's disease.

It is often difficult for family members to confront the patient about driving. This is particularly true if the patient relies on driving to perform day-to-day activities or attend social functions. If the healthy spouse does not drive, the entire family's mobility is disrupted. A discussion about the hazards of driving with the patient's health care provider (e.g. physician, nurse, social worker), the patient, and the family caregiver provides a forum to discuss this important issue.

In some regions it is required that the physician report the diagnosis of dementia to motor vehicle bureaus leading to cancellation of the patient's license. However, it is usually up to the family to make the decision. It should be remembered that a canceled driver's license will not necessarily prevent an Alzheimer's disease patient from driving. Sometimes families resort to trickery: changing car keys, or even disabling the car.

How does Alzheimer's disease affect personal care and grooming?

Personal care refers to dressing, bathing, shaving, toileting, eating, and maintaining one's appearance. Although these tasks seem straight forward, they involve complex functions of judgement, planning, and visuospatial skills. These activities are called basic activities of daily living (ADL).

Typically, patients with mild Alzheimer's disease show little impairment in their ADLs. In part, this is because these tasks are highly learned and repeated throughout one's life. Prompting the patient to wash or dress may be necessary at this stage, yet the Alzheimer's disease patient is still quite independent.

In the moderate stage of the illness, the patient has more difficulty performing ADLs. If unsupervised, the patient may choose clothes that do not complement one another or are inappropriate for the weather. Problems with the normal sequence of dressing may also occur: underwear may be put on over trousers. Buttoning or closing a belt may be difficult and require assistance. In order to lessen difficulties with dressing, it may be helpful to simplify choices available to the Alzheimer's disease patient. Clothes that are easy to put on, like warm up suits and slip on shoes, can also be quite useful.

Bathing and showering usually need some supervision in the moderate stage because the Alzheimer's disease patient is at risk of scalding with hot water and may have difficulty drying adequately. Shaving with an electric razor may be a good alternative to using traditional blades since it does not require use of the faucet or sharp blades. Alzheimer's disease patients

SYMPTOMS ASSOCIATED WITH MILD, MODERATE, AND SEVERE STAGES OF ALZHEIMER'S DISEASE

Cognitive/ Functional Domain	Mild Stage	Moderate Stage	Severe Stage
Memory	Consistent memory loss; more prominent for recent events	Severe memory loss; only highly learned material retained	Severe memory loss only fragments remain
Orientation	Moderate difficulty with time relationships; may be disoriented to place	Severe difficulty with time relationships; usually disoriented to time, often to place	Oriented to person only
Problem Solving	Mild difficulty handling problems; social judgment usually maintained	Severely impaired in handling problems; social judgement usually impaired	Unable to make judgements or solve problems
Community Affairs	Impairment in these activities, though may be engaged in some	Unable to independently function outside the home	Unable to independently function outside of home, appears too ill to be taken to functions outside the home
Home and Hobbies	Mild impairment of function at home; more difficult chores, hobbies, and interests impaired	Only simple chores preserved; impaired ability to sustain interest in activities	No significant function in the home
Personal Care	Needs prompting	Requires assistance in dressing, grooming, keeping of personal effects	Requires much assistance with personal care

Figure 6.2 *Lists the symptoms across several cognitive and functional domains that are observed in the different stages of Alzheimer's disease. These groupings serve as guidance and can vary substantially among different individuals. As adapted from Hughes et al, 1982.*

metimes prefer, or demand, to always wear the same clothes, event to
d for sleep. The caregiver can use bath time as an opportunity to
place the worn clothes with a fresh set. Purchase of duplicate outfits
ty be necessary. Brushing teeth and combing hair may or may not
quire direct assistance. Incontinence can occur at this stage and can be
anaged with adult diapers and a regular toileting schedule. Maintenance
good hygiene is very important, but is sometimes overlooked in patients
th Alzheimer's disease.

the severe stage of the illness, patients need supervision and assistance
th all ADLs. Complete assistance with bathing, grooming, and toileting is
quired at this stage. Dressing the Alzheimer's disease patient in clothes
at are easy to put on can lessen the frustration with this activity. The
tient will be unable to cut food, and may need to be fed. A synopsis of
e various changes in cognition and functioning are listed, according to
ness severity, in Figure 6.2. Since patients with Alzheimer's disease
rtainly vary in terms of the symptoms they demonstrate, Figure 6.2
ould serve only as a working framework, rather than a precise guide.

What behavioral changes occur in Alzheimer's disease?

ttients with Alzheimer's disease often experience behavioral disturbances
some point during the course of the illness. These symptoms, termed
oncognitive disturbances, can occur at any stage of the illness. Behavioral
isturbances wax and wane in their intensity and vary widely from person
person. These behaviors may cause significant distress for the patient,
nd burden for the family caregiver. The symptoms can be treated either
rith environmental techniques or medication. Early recognition,
nderstanding, and management of these behaviors can improve the
uality of life for both Alzheimer's disease patients and their caregivers.

What mood changes occur in Alzheimer's disease?

amily members often comment that the Alzheimer's disease patient
ppears depressed, with decreased interest in doing things. It is important
o ask the Alzheimer's disease patient about his/her mood and desire to
articipate in activities. Social withdrawal may be a manifestation of
ognitive impairment (as described above), but may be aggravated by
lepressed mood. However, it is important to note that patients with severe

Alzheimer's disease may not be able to report their mood because of language difficulties. If depression is being considered in a patient with Alzheimer's disease, the full constellation of symptoms of depression must be assessed. These include the presence of depressed mood (or frequent crying) and/or decreased interest in most things. In addition, the patient should be assessed for the following symptoms: decreased energy, change in appetite or weight loss, sleep disturbance, low self-esteem or guilt, decreased concentration, and thoughts of suicide or that life is not worth living. If the patient has at least five of the above symptoms nearly everyday, most of the day, for at least two weeks, he/she may have a diagnosis of clinical depression. An antidepressant medication should definitely be considered in this situation. There is less consensus regarding the usefulness of medications for individuals with fewer symptoms, or with less pervasive presentation of these symptoms. Physicians make these decisions on a case-by-case basis.

It is important that clinicians understand the relationship between Alzheimer's disease and depression. The terms pseudo-dementia and dementia syndrome of depression have been applied to patients who present primarily complaining of memory loss but who have an underlying depression. Older persons who experience memory loss should undergo a full evaluation for mood disorder prior to being given the diagnosis of Alzheimer's disease. Depression may be distinguished from Alzheimer's disease on the basis of the following: 1) Alzheimer's disease usually is not complicated by a depression with the all the symptoms stated above, 2) depression usually has a shorter time course (more rapid onset), and 3) a past history of depression suggests that the patient may be experiencing a recurrence of an underlying depressive disorder. If the diagnosis is unclear, the patient should be treated appropriately for a depression, followed by re-evaluation of cognitive deficits. Patients who have both Alzheimer's disease and depression should also be treated for depression.

What personality changes occur in Alzheimer's disease?

Patients with Alzheimer's disease often experience personality changes. A common example is irritability: the patient may become very angry or lose his/her temper without clear provocation. Patients may also develop socially inappropriate behavior. The behavioral disturbances are unpredictable, and can develop in patients who were very calm prior to the illness. Conversely, an individual who was formerly very gregarious and outgoing may become quiet and socially withdrawn. Because of his/her memory deficit, the Alzheimer's disease patient may have no awareness of these personality changes and may deny them upon confrontation.

What perceptual changes occur in Alzheimer's disease?

Perceptions refer to an individual's beliefs about the reality of events, and sensory observations of environmental stimuli. A delusion refers to a fixed false belief that is not consistent with the environmental reality. A hallucination refers to visual, auditory, olfactory, or tactile perceptions that are experienced in the absence of external stimuli. Patients with Alzheimer's disease may experience either of these perceptual disturbances, alone or in combination.

Often an Alzheimer's disease patient's delusion can be understood in the context of the cognitive changes that occur in the illness. It is not uncommon for an Alzheimer's disease patient to misplace objects and query others about their whereabouts. Sometimes, these concerns escalate until the Alzheimer's disease patient has the paranoid delusion that someone has stolen objects such as money, jewelry, clothes, and car keys. The Alzheimer's disease patient may accuse their loved ones of stealing from them and become quite agitated about these concerns.

Alzheimer's disease patients may believe that family members who have moved out or are deceased are living in the house. The patient may also state that strangers or neighbors have moved in. These beliefs may be confused with visual hallucinations in which the patient actually sees these inhabitants. The belief that family members are once again living in the house can be quite unshakable, despite clear evidence to the contrary. Paranoid delusions about strangers can relate to the fears the Alzheimer's disease patient has about things being stolen. At times, there is no way to understand these beliefs other than in the context of biological brain changes that accompany Alzheimer's disease.

Management of delusions must be determined on a case by case basis. Calm reassurance about the reality of the situation (reality testing) may alleviate the concern temporarily. However, the delusion can recur in spite of repeated reassurances. Confrontation should be avoided. At times, caregivers find that the best course of action is to ignore or "play along with" mistaken beliefs. Changes to the environment should be avoided; placement of objects in the same place at all times may be helpful. Delusions that are infrequent, amenable to reality testing, or are not distressful may only require the above caregiver interventions. If these delusions cause distress for the Alzheimer's disease patient and/or the caregiver, appropriate management by a physician may be quite helpful (see section on treatment of behavioral disturbance below).

The distinction between a delusion that someone is in the home and the visual hallucination that people are there may be difficult. Overall, hallucinations are much less frequent than delusions in Alzheimer's disease. If an Alzheimer's disease patient has a visual impairment, visual hallucinations may be more likely to occur. In such a case, specific treatment of the visual deficit, for example with cataract extraction, will be beneficial. As with delusions, hallucinations may not require treatment with medication if they are not distressing to the patient or the caregiver.

Does agitation occur in Alzheimer's disease?

Agitation refers to a constellation of behaviors, including verbally aggressive behavior and physical agitation. When these behaviors worsen in the evening and night, the term "sun-downing" is given; the result can be sleep-deprivation for the Alzheimer's disease patient and the caregiver. A physician consultation may be quite helpful for medication management of these behaviors. These symptoms often cause significant caregiver burden.

Examples of verbally aggressive behavior include yelling or cursing. The individual may repeatedly say the same things, without any clear provocation. These symptoms can be quite disruptive to the environment, especially if they are continuous for any period of time.

Alzheimer's disease patients also may display increased pacing and decreased ability to sit calmly. Aimless wandering into different rooms sometimes is accompanied by rummaging through drawers, an activity that can at times be problematic. The optimal management of this behavior is to adjust the house so that the patient cannot wander into dangerous areas (e.g. tool rooms) or gain access to unlocked cabinets. Chastising the patient for these behaviors is usually not of much help. Redirection to other activities or tolerance of wandering (when safety is assured) is usually most beneficial.

BEHAVIORAL SYMPTOMS OBSERVED IN ALZHEIMER'S DISEASE

◆ Mood changes: depression, apathy, tearfulness, low self-esteem

◆ Personality changes: irritability, social inappropriateness, withdrawal

◆ Agitation: verbal or physical aggression, pacing, restlessness

◆ Perceptual changes: paranoia, delusions, hallucinations

◆ Sleep changes: increased or decreased sleep

◆ Appetite changes: diminished or increased appetite, craving for sweets

Figure 6.3 *Lists some of the behavioral symptoms that may occur in Alzheimer's disease.*

The Alzheimer's disease patient may only exhibit verbally or physically aggressive behavior upon caregiving, including bathing, grooming, and meal times. Some of these behaviors may reflect the patient's frustration with the inability to do these tasks or a lack of comprehension of their purpose. Consistent and predictable routines with ample time allotment and reasonable expectations on the part of the caregiver may improve these behaviors. Different approaches, including changing the timing of these activities and increased caregiver involvement, may also improve the experience. Figure 6.3 lists the most common behavioral disturbances observed in Alzheimer's disease.

What is the course of Alzheimer's disease symptoms?

The course of the Alzheimer's disease can range between 3 and 14 years from the time of diagnosis until death. Patients have usually been experiencing symptoms for 2 to 3 years prior to the time of their initial evaluation with a physician. Memory and judgment/problem solving impairments are usually the earliest signs. Difficulties in orientation and ADLs are typically later developments. Behavioral symptoms are more variable and episodic than cognitive symptoms; their relationship with illness severity is therefore not as predictable.

ALZHEIMER'S DISEASE

CHAPTER 7

ALZHEIMER'S DISEASE AND THE CAREGIVER

Elizabeth Fine and Deborah B. Marin

What is meant by the term caregiver?

A caregiver is an individual who contributes to the care of a patient with Alzheimer's disease. The primary caregiver is the individual who is ultimately responsible for the Alzheimer's patient's well-being. Usually the spouse or daughter of the affected individual takes on this very important role. Because caring for an Alzheimer's patient can be very stressful, caregivers need to learn techniques that aid them in the caregiving process. They also should know about support systems which can be invaluable for their own quality of life, as well as the well-being of the patient. Informal supports refer to unpaid help, including friends and family. Formal supports include professional healthcare providers (e.g. physicians, nurses, social workers), paid home healthcare attendants, various day programs, and residential facilities.

What happens if there is no one who can be the caregiver?

The Alzheimer's disease patient in all likelihood cannot arrange for the appropriate supports to ensure his/her well-being. In part, this is due to the fact that Alzheimer's disease patients often are not aware of the extent of their cognitive problems. If there is no available primary caregiver to supervise the patient, a family member may rely on health care providers for arrangement of appropriate caregiving services. These health care providers include social workers, nurses, physicians, or community based organizations (senior centers or religious organizations). If there are adequate financial resources, a home attendant may be hired. Assisted living facilities are potential alternatives for living arrangements as well. If the Alzheimer's patient has significant medical illness and/or requires skilled nursing, a chronic care facility may be appropriate.

If there is no family member to arrange for the above services and the patient is unsafe on his/her own, the healthcare provider may arrange for a court-appointed guardian. The guardian will work with the health care provider to arrange for appropriate care. In the absence of a guardian, the health care provider may contact Protective Services for Adults in order to place the individual into a safe environment. The telephone number of your local Protective Services for Adults is listed in the phone directory.

What is the range of caregiving tasks?

Alzheimer's disease affects all areas of cognition and functioning. Consequently the caregiving tasks can be far-reaching (see Figure 7.1). Because of the evolving nature of the illness, the caregiver role changes over time. Caregiving tasks include acting as the patient's advocate, assisting with day-to-day activities, and providing psychological support. If the caregiver is a spouse, many of these tasks are a continuation of an existing relationship. However, for many caregivers, these tasks represent new and very different responsibilities. If there is no spouse to be the primary caregiver, the adult daughter often assumes the primary caregiving role. Below is a description of caregiving tasks, and their relationship to the different stages of Alzheimer's disease.

Beginning in the mild stage of the illness, the caregiver must assess the need for adequate supervision to ensure the patient's safety. In the mild stage, the Alzheimer's disease patient does not necessarily need to be supervised throughout the day. If the patient does not have a problem

---

RANGE OF CAREGIVER TASKS

◆ Providing or arranging for adquate supervision

◆ Ensuring medical well-being of the patient

◆ Arranging for financial security of the patient

◆ Assisting with household chores

◆ Assisting with personal care

◆ Providing support and companionship

Figure 7.1 *Lists major tasks for a family doctor member or paid individual who cares for an Alzheimer's individual. The amount of care required depends on the level of functioning of the individual with the illness.*

with orientation, he/she may be able to be on his/her own for a period of time each day. Daily visits and phone calls are still necessary to check on the patient's well being. Even the patient with mild impairments is at risk of getting lost, causing household floods, leaving the stove on too long, or being flustered by household emergencies. Each situation needs to be evaluated before determination of the correct amount of caregiver supervision is made.

The mild Alzheimer's disease patient may also requires help with finances. He/she can be a target for financial scams, forget to pay bills, withdraw inappropriately large sums of money from the bank, and forget to deposit monthly checks. It is therefore necessary for caregivers to consult with an Elder Care attorney and financial advisor to make financial arrangements for the future.

In the mild stage, the Alzheimer's disease patient may be able to continue to do most household chores, including meal preparation and cleaning. Shopping may be more affected because it requires leaving the home and handling money.

In the moderate stage, caregivers need to arrange for significant supervision of the Alzheimer's disease patient. The affected individual should not be left on his/her own at this stage since he/she is very likely to be disoriented to time and place. Since the Alzheimer's patient can no longer handle money and is at risk of getting lost, the caregiver has to arrange all errands and appointments, including shopping, going to social engagements, and visits to the doctor. In the moderate stage, the Alzheimer's disease patient is more likely to requires assistance with grooming, dressing, and possibly toileting. He/she needs to be reminded when to eat meals and to go to bed. Providing reassurance and reducing confusion become part of the caregiver's responsibilities.

When the Alzheimer's disease patient reaches the severe stage of the illness, he/she requires total care. In addition to providing constant supervision and conducting all household tasks, the caregiver must feed, bathe, dress, and toilet the affected individual.

Caregivers often note the importance of providing psychological support for the Alzheimer's disease patient throughout the illness. The caregiver often becomes the only social contact for the Alzheimer's disease patient since friends and family members may withdraw as the disease progresses.

Caregivers find themselves educating friends and family about the illness in order to maintain relationships for themselves and the Alzheimer's disease patient.

How stressful is caregiving?

The caregiving process can be very stressful. Caregivers of Alzheimer's disease patients often experience caregiver burden that manifests itself in psychological, financial, and physical domains. Typical responses of the caregiver to the caregiving process are listed in Figure 7.2. The psychological reactions observed in caregivers may include anxiety, depression, irritability, anger, sleep disturbances, and fatigue. Caregivers may experience guilt about the adequacy of their caregiving, in spite of tremendous efforts on their part. Anger about the illness and toward the Alzheimer's patient may also occur. Family members may also worry about the safety of the Alzheimer's patient or about how they will provide adequate care. Caregivers may turn to prescription or over-the-counter sedatives or alcohol to medicate some of these symptoms.

Caregiving often requires major role shifts which can be very stressful. For example, wives who relied on their husbands for all financial matters may have to learn these skills for the first time in their lives. Husbands may have to learn how to cook and manage the house. Children who relied on their parents for security and support find themselves in a parenting role. Adjustment to these role changes can be quite difficult.

The social consequences of caregiving include family conflicts, decreased life satisfaction, and social isolation. Caregivers may hide the diagnosis from friends because they fear the social stigma associated with the illness

---

TYPICAL RESPONSES TO THE CAREGIVING PROCESS

◆ Guilt   ◆ Anxiety   ◆ Depression

◆ Anger   ◆ Fatigue   ◆ Sleep disturbances

◆ Financial Strain ◆ Role strain   ◆ Social isolation

◆ Satisfaction

Figure 7.2 *Lists some, but not all, experiences of caregivers for individuals with Alzheimer's disease. Although many of the responses may reflect burden, caregivers often derive satisfaction from the role of caring.*

They may withdraw from social interactions because they do not want their loved one to suffer embarrassment.

Caring for an Alzheimer's patient is very expensive. Since caregivers spend on average 7-14 hours per day in the caregiving process, the annual cost of time spent caregiving is very high. The economic consequences are particularly devastating for family members who must forego working in order to care for their ill relative. Home attendants are also very costly, and are not covered by most insurance policies.

Caregivers often neglect their own health. They may not exercise adequately or keep doctors' appointments because they cannot leave their relative with Alzheimer's disease. Caring for an Alzheimer's patient may be physically taxing, especially for an older individual who has physical ailments. If the patient has a sleep disturbance, the caregiver may not get enough sleep either.

The extent of caregiver burden is influenced by several factors. Individuals have different methods of coping with stress. A caregiver with a coping style that includes a take-charge, problem-solving attitude may experience less stress. The quality of the relationship between the caregiver and the Alzheimer's disease patient prior to onset of the illness may affect the amount of burden experienced by the caregiver. A pre-existing strained relationship may become substantially worse.

The severity of the Alzheimer's disease patient's behavioral disturbances and cognitive impairment can also affect the amount of burden experienced by the caregiver. Alzheimer's disease patients may become more confused and agitated in the evening and at night, often depriving the caregiver of rest. Consultation with a clinician may be quite helpful for management of these behaviors.

It must be remembered that caregiver stress is not a reflection of weakness. Rather, this reaction reflects the complexity and strain of the caregiving process. Conversely, caregivers may experience satisfaction in their role, knowing that they are doing their best in providing care for the Alzheimer's patient.

ALZHEIMER'S DISEASE

What methods can enhance the well being of the caregiver and the Alzheimer's disease patient?

Caregiving can be an all encompassing experience. It is essential that caregivers learn various strategies that enhance their ability to care for the Alzheimer's patient. This section will review caregiving techniques and services that can decrease caregiver burden and enhance the well-being of the Alzheimer's disease patient (See Figure 7.3).

Alzheimer's patients respond very favorably to predictable events and structure. A regular routine that involves a set time for meals, errands, recreational activities, and personal care can be invaluable. Most caregivers find that trying to do the job alone is an impossible undertaking. Enlisting the help of family and friends as well as healthcare professionals (as described below) can help to ease the burden. It is important for the caregiver to have time set aside in the day to socialize with friends, make medical appointments, and care for the house and finances. Personal time can involve such things as watching television, listening to music, or having coffee with friends.

How can the Alzheimer's Association be helpful?

The Alzheimer's Association is a national non-profit organization that provides a wide range of information and services to Alzheimer's disease

---

METHODS TO ENHANCE CAREGIVER WELL-BEING

◆ Develop a daily schedule

◆ Set aside time for yourself

◆ Coordinate caregiving among different family members and friends

◆ Engage in relaxing activities on a daily basis

◆ Attend a support group or individual counseling

◆ Maintain a social network

◆ Hire professional caregiver to help when necessary

◆ Consider day programs to long-term care placement if appropriate

---

Figure 7.3 *Lists some techniques that are helpful for reducing caregiver stress.*

patients and their friends and family members. The telephone number of the national office in the US is (312) 881-8008. Each state has a local chapter that is listed in the local phone directory and most countries have listings in their city telephone directories. The Alzheimer's Association has regular educational seminars covering the diagnosis, clinical presentation, and treatment of Alzheimer's disease, research options available, legal and financial planning, methods to hire and evaluate home health care attendants, and nursing home placement. Seminars also teach techniques to cope with the diagnosis and manage cognitive and behavioral changes. Each Alzheimer's Association chapter can provide a list of healthcare providers who are experts in the diagnosis and treatment of the illness. Typically, each chapter also offers support groups for family members and friends of Alzheimer's disease patients. The Alzheimer's Association, which also supports research efforts, is an invaluable resource.

What are caregiver support groups?

Support groups are an excellent resource to help the caregiver cope with Alzheimer's disease. The groups offer education about Alzheimer's disease, provide social networks, and offer a safe and accepting environment in which caregivers can share their reactions to the illness. In support groups, caregivers share methods to manage the cognitive impairment and problem behaviors. Many caregivers find that support groups successfully combat the social isolation that they often experience. However, groups are not for everyone. Each person deals with being a caregiver differently, and some are not comfortable with participation in this type of forum.

Support groups may be set up for spouses or adult children, or mixed groups for both spouses and extended family and friends. The groups may meet weekly to monthly. Support groups are led by either a healthcare provider (social worker, registered nurse, psychologist) or by a lay person who is a caregiver. The Alzheimer's Association has training sessions for those who are interested in leading a support group. To join a group, contact your local chapter of the Alzheimer's Association for a referral.

Are there support groups for the Alzheimer patient?

In the early stages of the illness, Alzheimer's disease patients may benefit from a support group and/or individual counseling, just as it has been shown that patients suffering from other chronic illnesses benefit from group therapy. There are a growing number of this type of support group across the country. Your local chapter of the Alzheimer's Association will know the availability of such groups in you area.

How can individual or family counseling help?

Alzheimer's disease is an illness that takes a heavy toll on the primary caregiver and the entire family. The emotional and physical strain may bring family members together, or conversely increase tensions. Counselors and therapists can help individual family members or the family as a group cope with caring for a patient with Alzheimer's disease.

What are geriatric care managers?

Geriatric care managers counsel caregivers with legal and financial issues, arrange for home health attendants and provide supportive therapy to help families cope with caring for a patient with Alzheimer's disease. They are usually social workers or nurse practitioners who have worked in the field of geriatrics. There is a national association of Professional Geriatric Care Managers in the US that can be reached at (602) 881-8008 for local referrals.

What do paid home health attendants do?

Paid home health attendants provide a wide range of services. In the mild stage of Alzheimer's disease the home health attendant is needed primarily for the supervision of the Alzheimer's disease patient. This can include accompanying the patient to appointments, movies or other activities. As the illness progresses the home health attendant can assist the patient with ADLs, e.g. bathing, dressing, eating, and toileting. The paid attendants also provide assistance with household responsibilities such as cooking, shopping and laundry.

When is it time to hire a home health attendant?

This is one of the most difficult things for a family caregiver to determine, partly because it represents an admission that the Alzheimer's disease patient has lost independence. Many families feel guilty that they are unable to provide the care that is required. However, it is essential that a home health attendant be considered as soon as the safety of the Alzheimer's disease patient is in question. Often, family members believe that they should be completely responsible for care for their relative. This is absolutely not the right choice for everyone.

Family members may fear that the patient will not accept home care. Caregivers are, appropriately, aware that they are interfering with the patient's self determination. Because the Alzheimer's patient may not have the capacity to evaluate his/her own needs, family members may have to override the resistance. Actually, providing a home attendant does preserve the patient's autonomy since it may delay placement in a chronic care facility. Often, the patient willingly accepts the help once the attendant is in place.

Who covers the cost of home health attendants?

The cost of home health attendants is predominantly paid by the family. In the US, Medicare does pay for home health attendants for a limited period of time if an Alzheimer's disease patient has medical problems that interfere with bathing, dressing, toileting or preparing meals. The number of hours provided by Medicare, as well as the duration of this service, vary depending on the patient's medical situation and the state in which he/she resides. If the Alzheimer's disease patient requires skilled nursing services as a result of concurrent medical problems, Medicare will provide a registered nurse for a limited period of time.

There are some insurance policies (long-term care policies) as well as some Health Maintenance Organizations that do cover the costs of home care attendant services, usually for a limited number of total hours. Some health plans cover home health attendants only for a limited time period following hospitalization.

Medicaid, a program for the poor or disabled, pays for the services of a home care attendant for a patient with Alzheimer's disease who has no medical problems. The number of hours covered by Medicaid varies significantly from state to state. Local chapters of the Alzheimer's Association can provide information about state Medicaid benefits. The application for Medicaid can be picked up at the Department of Social Services. Geriatric care managers, elder care attorneys and social workers in community based programs such as Catholic Charities can assist caregivers with this application procedure.

How does one go about hiring a home health attendant?

The are a large number of home healthcare agencies that be contacted to hire a home health attendant. The local Alzheimer's Association chapter can also provide guidance.

There are some less formal avenues to finding a home health attendant. One is to enquire at local religious organizations or community agencies such as Catholic Charities; some of these groups provide home care attendants. Frequently, caregivers find home health attendants through word of mouth. Recommendations are often provided by members of support groups. While there are no guarantees that the attendant will take good care of the Alzheimer's disease patient, the chances are better when the recommendation of a reputable agency or a personal contact is followed.

It is important that the home attendant is familiar with Alzheimer's disease, and preferably has had some formal training. An attendant who has been educated regarding dementia care and has practical experience will be best suited to deal with an Alzheimer's disease patient. You can ask the home care agency if they have trained their attendants. Specifically, you can enquire about their views on adequate training. Some Alzheimer's Association chapters and medical centers provide training for home attendants. Caregivers may be able to send their attendants to these training sessions.

Depending on the needs of the person with the illness, it is usually best to gradually increase the hours a health attendant works. This process enables the Alzheimer's disease patient to become accustomed to having someone new around the house. As the patient's needs increase, caregivers can increase the amount of time that the home attendant is utilized. Open communication between the caregiver and the attendant is critical. Review of the Alzheimer's patient's routines, likes, and dislikes is often very helpful. If the caregiver questions the quality of care that is being provided, these concerns should be discussed with the attendant and/or the home care agency. For those families who do not live near the Alzheimer's disease patient, a geriatric care manager can assist in hiring and supervising the home health attendant.

What are adult day programs?

Adult day programs provide an environment in which Alzheimer's disease patients participate in activities. These programs provide reminiscence groups, exercise classes, arts and crafts, music therapy, and meals. They provide respite for the caregivers and stimulation for the patient. Some of these programs provide medical screening. The medical model programs may be covered under Medicare as well as Medicaid, and may also accept paying clients. The social model day programs are not covered by Medicare. Adult day programs are found throughout the United States and can be associated with nursing homes or community-based organizations. The local chapter of the Alzheimer's Association or the Department of Aging can identify nearby programs.

Most adult day programs are geared toward Alzheimer's disease patients in the mild to moderate stage of the disease. When the patient is unable to be left alone for any period of time but still has the ability to socialize and enjoy activities (e.g. arts and crafts), he/she can benefit from this type of program.

How does one choose an adult day program?

Before bringing the Alzheimer's disease patient to an adult day program, the caregiver should visit the center alone. One should determine if there are other people in the program who are in a similar stage of the illness. The caregiver should make sure that there is a good staff-to-patient ratio (one staff/volunteer to four Alzheimer's disease patients), and observe the way that staff members interact with the patients. Inquiries can be made about transportation services. These programs may be open from three to twelve hours a day, and some are open seven days a week. Alzheimer's disease patients initially attend adult day programs once or twice a week, depending on the needs of the patient and the caregiver. It will generally take the Alzheimer's disease patient a number of visits before he/she becomes familiar with the program. For this reason, it is usually a good idea for the caregiver to accompany the patient for the first few sessions.

Are there other forms of respite services?

There are inpatient respite programs that are affiliated with nursing homes, and independent community-based respite facilities. These facilities generally provide up to three weeks of respite to families. Most of these services are not covered by insurance, except Medicaid. Names of these types of respite services are available by contacting your local chapter of the Alzheimer's Association or the Department of Aging.

When should one consider respite programs?

Respite programs can be used for emergency situations when the caregiver is suddenly unable to care for the Alzheimer's disease patient. They can also be used when caregivers feel they need a rest from the caregiving role. Unfortunately, some caregivers feel that time off is a luxury rather than a necessity. Also, these programs are very time-limited and may not be readily available.

What other community based programs are available to assist caregivers?

Meals on Wheels services are available to individuals over 65 years of age. For a nominal fee, Meals on Wheels delivers two meals a day, usually six days a week, to the individual's home. This can assist the caregiver with the often burdensome task of meal preparation.

There are a number of volunteer organizations that may be available locally to provide some assistance with housekeeping services for older adults. Information about such services can be obtained in the US from Elder Care Locators, (800) 677-1116.

What is the role of assisted living facilities?

Over the past few years, there has been significant growth in the number of residential facilities that provide several services for older adults. For example, these environments may provide meals, activities, housekeeping, and a social environment in which to meet people. Some places also provide on-site nursing and medical services. These facilities are not federally regulated like nursing homes. As a consequence, it is important for the consumer to review the safety of the environment for Alzheimer's patients. Depending on the facility and the patient, these living arrangements may be reasonable for Alzheimer's patients in the mild stage of the illness. One can enquire whether the facility has an alternative setting for individuals who require more care or supervision.

What is the role of nursing homes?

A nursing home is a facility that a person enters when he/she is no longer able to be cared for in his/her own home. The nursing home provides twenty-four hour nursing care and supervision. All nursing homes provide certain basic services such as recreational activities, bathing, grooming, meals, medical and nursing care. Nursing homes vary in the specific activities they provide, ranging from special groups for patients with Alzheimer's disease, to pet therapy programs, and trips out in the community. There are an increasing number of dementia care units in nursing homes, with specially trained staff and therapeutic programs.

Nursing homes may be owned by state/local governments (public nursing homes), individuals, corporations, religious or charitable organizations. Nursing homes are either not-for-profit (voluntary nursing homes), or for profit (proprietary nursing homes). There are federal and state standards that govern the operation of all nursing homes.

When is it time to consider nursing home placement?

The decision to move the Alzheimer's disease patient into a nursing home is rarely made easily. There is no specific time when someone must be placed in a nursing home. The decision is based on the individual circumstances of each Alzheimer's disease patient and his/her family. If an Alzheimer's disease patient lives alone in the community without friends or family to provide supervision, a nursing home may be the safest place to reside. If the patient has been cared for at home with the help of a home attendant and a network of family and friends, the decision to place someone in a nursing home is more complicated.

Incontinence and the need for significant personal care are common reasons for nursing home placement. Financial considerations can also favor placement. The Alzheimer's disease patient may develop behaviors that are considered unmanageable at home. Of all the predictors of placement, behavioral disturbances are most treatable. Proper consultation with a physician, especially a geriatric psychiatrist, may result in medication management that improves difficult behaviors. If the safety of the Alzheimer's disease patient or the caregiver is in question, or if the Alzheimer's disease patient has additional medical problems requiring skilled care, placement in a nursing home may be the best option.

It is important to remember that the caregiver can significantly enhance the experience of an individual in a nursing home. This outcome can be accomplished by regular visits, and open communication with the patient's healthcare providers.

How does one choose a nursing home?

Selecting a nursing home can be a difficult and often time-consuming endeavor. Friends, family members, physicians, nurses, and social workers can provide recommendations. The caregiver should set up appointments to visit each nursing home under consideration. The evaluation should include the following questions: Is it clean? How is medical care provided? How do the staff relate to the patients? Is there a good staff-to-patient ratio? Is there a special Alzheimer's unit? How often are physical restraints used? Are patients' personal belongings in the rooms? What are the visiting hours? What is the availability of ethnic foods or special dietary preferences? What is the policy on taking patients out of the facility for short visits with family or friends? It is important that the nursing home be located near to the members of the family and friends who will be visiting. After choosing the most desirable nursing homes, the caregiver should place the Alzheimer's disease patient on the waiting lists; most homes are generally kept at full capacity.

How does one know if the nursing home is taking good care of the Alzheimer's disease patient?

While all nursing homes are inspected annually to ensure that they meet federal standards, it is important for the caregiver to maintain an active presence, overseeing the care provided to the Alzheimer's disease patient. A good working relationship with the staff is important. There are usually monthly meetings between families and the nursing home staff that allow specific issues to be discussed. If a caregiver feels that a nursing home resident is not receiving appropriate care, the Ombudsman Program For Long-Term Care (listed in local US telephone directories) can be of assistance.

Who covers the cost of a nursing home?

The cost of nursing homes varies. In most US states, few people can afford to pay for a nursing home for very long. Many nursing home residents are or become reliant upon state and federal subsidies.

Medicare provides a limited period of nursing home coverage, usually 100 days. The cost of the first 20 days is covered 100%, and from day 21-100 Medicare covers all but $89.50 per day. For Medicare coverage, the person must enter a nursing home directly from a hospital, or within 30 days of hospital discharge, and must have medical problems requiring skilled nursing care. It is important to realize that most people with Alzheimer's disease do not require skilled nursing services.

Medicaid covers 100% of nursing home costs for those who are eligible. It is the only provider of long-term care to most people in nursing homes. A small minority of people can afford to pay for nursing homes privately. Others have long-term health insurance that will cover nursing home costs. A person with the means for self-pay has a better chance of getting into the nursing home of choice. It is important to talk to an elder care lawyer to discuss long-term care planning (see Chapter 12).

How does one make the home safe for the Alzheimer's disease patient?

Securing the Alzheimer's disease patient's safety is one of the major responsibilities of the caregiver. Alzheimer's disease patients are at significant risk of wandering out of their environment and becoming lost. Three techniques are very useful to prevent and manage this problem. Provision of appropriate supervision in the home is essential. "Alzheimer's proofing" the home is also helpful. This includes changing the locks so that the external doors require a key to open from inside. Alarms can be placed on door knobs. These latter methods should be used in conjunction with, and not instead of, appropriate caregiver supervision.

In spite of the best efforts, Alzheimer's disease patients may get lost. The "Safe Return" program, offered by the Alzheimer's Association, provides family members with techniques to locate Alzheimer's disease patients in the event they become lost. For a very low fee, the program provides an identification bracelet, necklace, clothing tags, and wallet cards that provide information on whom to contact if the Alzheimer's disease patient is located. All participants are entered into a confidential national database that is accessible by police and health care providers. Health care providers, police, and fire departments are knowledgeable about this program and provide assistance. The Alzheimer's Association also helps family members by placing public service announcements on radio and television describing the lost Alzheimer's disease patient.

How should one communicate with an Alzheimer's patient?

The Alzheimer's disease patient loses the ability to communicate as the illness progresses. Words lose their meaning and emotional expressions may become the primary means of communication. This in turn causes increased stress in the relationship between the Alzheimer's disease patient and the caregiver. At all stages in the illness it is important to remember the three "C's": calm, concise, consistent. Use of a calm voice to communicate with the patient is very reassuring. Caregivers should speak in short and concise sentences, and look the person directly in the eye. As the Alzheimer's disease patient becomes more impaired, he/she will have an easier time responding to questions that require yes and no answers. It will also help the Alzheimer's disease patient if the caregiver sets up a consistent routine for the patient to follow. Consistency lessens the confusion that the Alzheimer's disease patient experiences, and may help to limit some caregiver stress. Figure 7.4 summarizes techniques to enhance communication with the Alzheimer's patient.

In the mild stage of the illness, the Alzheimer's disease patient may have word-finding difficulties. Caregivers may calmly offer word suggestions if this approach does not upset the Alzheimer's disease patient. The patient may be very repetitious. It is important for caregivers to tolerate this behavior. Changing the subject may break repetitive questions. Frequently the Alzheimer's disease patient digresses during a conversation. Gentle redirection may be effective.

The Alzheimer's disease patient may on occasion exhibit angry or tearful outbursts. These behaviors may be due in part to the frustration that he/she is experiencing. It is important that the caregiver not take these behaviors personally. The caregiver should try to determine the cause of

---

ENHANCING COMMUNICATION WITH ALZHEIMER'S INDIVIDUAL

◆ Use a calm voice to communicate with the individual

◆ Use short and concise sentences

◆ Create a consistent daily routine

◆ Be tolerent of repetitive questions or behavior

◆ Redirect rather than confront the individual

◆ Continue to engage in and shae pleasurable activities

Figure 7.4 *Lists techniques to enhance communication between caregivers and Alzheimer's individuals.*

the frustration, and try to diffuse the situation. Reassurance can be very calming. Comforting the Alzheimer's disease patient with kind words such as, "I'm here with you now, you don't have to worry"" often eases some of the fear that he/she is experiencing.

If hallucinations or delusions occur but do not seem to be upsetting to the patient, it is often best to avoid confrontation. The caregiver can provide calm reassurance that everything is alright and then change the topic. However if the hallucinations are distressing, the caregiver should contact the physician to discuss other treatment options. A significant and sudden change in behavior may reflect an emerging medical problem that the Alzheimer's disease patient is unable to communicate. The caregiver should contact the physician if this is a possibility.

In the later stages of the illness, the patient's verbal and emotional communication skills are increasingly impaired. The caregiver should use the sense of touch as a tool of communication. While verbal communication may be of limited value, caregivers can still share time with the patient by listening to music, looking at photographs, or just holding hands.

What activities are recommended with Alzheimer's disease patients?

The caregiver should try to continue activities enjoyed in the past with the Alzheimer's disease patient. Traditional hobbies such as gardening, painting, drawing, card games, scrabble, and puzzles are well received by Alzheimer's disease patients. Music has a wonderfully positive affect. Some people do volunteer work together, with the caregiver loosely supervising the Alzheimer's disease patient. Reminiscence therapy may also be very stimulating and rewarding. This involves looking at photographs, listening to music from the past, and remembering shared events.

ALZHEIMER'S DISEASE

CHAPTER 8

TREATING THE COGNITIVE SYMPTOMS

Is Alzheimer's disease treatable?

Until recently, Alzheimer's disease was considered to be an untreatable disease. Physicians learned in medical school that no medication improves memory, and that no treatment alters the course of the illness; for this reason, the attitude of clinicians toward individuals with the disease has often been fatalistic. Thankfully, the situation has changed. In the past few years, it has been proven that medication can augment cognitive function in patients with Alzheimer's disease, and there is evidence that the disease course can be modified. In addition, some of the behavioral dysfunction such as agitation, paranoia, and sleeplessness are readily treatable. Because of the recent success in the development of treatments for Alzheimer's disease, many medical schools and pharmaceutical companies are devoting major efforts to the discovery of more effective therapy. The outlook is good.

What can be done to improve a patient's memory?

The core cognitive symptoms of Alzheimer's disease are the inability to learn new information, problems with language, particularly finding words, and difficulty understanding spatial relationships. The class of drugs known as acetyl cholinesterase inhibitors increases the brain's concentrations of acetylcholine by inhibiting the enzyme, acetyl cholinesterase, that breaks down acetylcholine. Donepezil and tacrine, two drugs of this type, have been approved for the treatment of Alzheimer's disease cognitive symptoms, having been proven to be significantly better than placebo in treating these symptoms. In addition, rivastigmine has been approved in Europe, as has galanthamine in Austria. Both drugs are likely to be available soon in the United States.

The demonstration of statistically significant benefit in a controlled clinical trial does not necessarily mean that the benefit of a drug is clinically important. For this reason, the Food and Drug Administration received the advice of a special group to determine appropriate guidelines for the approval of drugs to treat Alzheimer's disease. It was established that the efficacy of a candidate drug must be shown not only on the psychometric tests that measure the core cognitive symptoms of Alzheimer's disease, but also on a measure of global status that can be scored by the clinician. All drugs approved for the treatment of Alzheimer's disease in the United States and Europe meet these standards.

What is an appropriate expectation for the cognitive effects of cholinesterase inhibitors?

Alzheimer's disease is a progressive disease; all patients suffer continuing decline in cognitive function. Patients who respond to cholinesterase inhibitors may, for a meaningful period of time, maintain or even improve cognitive function.

Some patients do not respond to inhibition of acetyl cholinesterase, and do no better with medication than with placebo. However, for others cholinesterase inhibitors produce clinically identifiable changes in memory language, orientation, attention or all of these cognitive areas. An apparent attenuation in the degree of decline over time may also be an indication of a favorable response.

With donepezil, improvement on cognitive testing can be observed within the first month of treatment. However, studies with these agents suggest that patient should remain on therapy for at least 3 months to fully assess the benefits of treatment. By 12 weeks of treatment, patients who receive either 5 or 10 mg/day of donepezil perform significantly better than patients who receive placebo. Often the therapeutic effects of tacrine are not apparent until patients are at a relatively high dose of the drug, 120 mg or 160 mg per day, and patients do not reach this dose until they have been receiving the drug for 12 to 18 weeks.

Why does it take so long to reach these upper doses of tacrine?

The administration of tacrine has been associated with an elevation in liver transaminases. These liver enzyme elevations suggest that the drug is stressing liver cells. Consequently, the treating physician must monitor liver enzyme levels, and adjust the treatment if there are significant abnormalities. By increasing the dose of tacrine very slowly, liver enzyme elevations can be somewhat minimized.

When such elevations occur, it does not mean that tacrine therapy cannot still be a part of a patient's treatment regimen. Rather, it means that the dose must be reduced or discontinued, and eventually the patient restarted at a lower dose, and titrated to a higher dose more slowly. Thus, the use of tacrine requires great patience on the part of caregiver, physician, and Alzheimer's patient.

How do donepezil and tacrine compare?

There are no clinical studies that directly compare the two medications. When comparing the higher doses of tacrine to donepezil, the results on cognitive testing appear similar.

Donepezil is a once a day medication, whereas tacrine is given in divided doses four times a day. A scheduled dose increase is required for tacrine, as is blood monitoring on a bi-weekly basis during dose titration because of the need to follow liver function tests. Donepezil is started at 5 mg/day and may be increased to 10 mg/day after 4-6 weeks; no blood test monitoring is required with donepezil. The efficacy of tacrine is most likely to be observed at the 120 or 160 mg/day dose. The higher dose of 10 mg/day of donepezil does not provide a statistically greater clinical benefit than 5 mg, but there is a suggestion that the higher dose may provide additional benefits for some patients.

As noted above, tacrine can have adverse effects on the liver; donepezil, on the other hand, does not cause liver toxicity. Both medications produce side effects that include nausea, diarrhea, insomnia, fatigue, and anorexia. The higher doses of these medications are associated with an increased rate of these effects. The side effects seem to be less severe and less frequent with donepezil than the higher doses of tacrine. With donepezil, taking the lower dose (5 mg/day) for 4-6 weeks before increasing to 10 mg/day minimizes the side effects at the higher dose.

Many patients who begin treatment with tacrine are not able to continue the medication. Because donepezil is easier to use and is not associated with liver toxicity, most patients are able to continue treatment with this medication.

As a result of these advantages, since the approval of donepezil there is little use of tacrine as a treatment for the cognitive deficits of Alzheimer's disease.

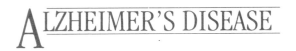

Are other drugs besides donepezil and tacrine in development?

The pharmaceutical industry is working aggressively and rapidly to develop other cholinesterase inhibitors. Some of these agents may even be more efficacious than donepezil or tacrine. Galanthamine is a cholinesterase inhibitor currently marketed in Austria for the treatment of Alzheimer's disease; rivastigmine is another such drug recently approved in Europe. Metrifonate, also a drug in this class, is currently under review by the FDA.

Are there other approaches to increased cholinergic activity?

It is theoretically possible to increase acetylcholine activity by several avenues; inhibition of the enzyme that breaks down acetylcholine, acetyl cholinesterase, is only one such approach. Others include increasing the release of acetylcholine, and direct stimulation of receptors for acetylcholine. The latter approach has received a great deal of attention; the class of drugs called muscarinic agonists increase cholinergic activity in the brain by binding to acetylcholine receptors. Ultimately, clinical trials will tell whether this approach is more or less effective than cholinesterase inhibition. Unfortunately, to date most of the large scale studies have shown that these products are not well tolerated at the doses needed to show a benefit, nor have they demonstrated the efficacy of cholinesterase inhibitors..

CHAPTER 9

TREATING THE DISEASE PROCESS

Are there drugs that may stop the progression of Alzheimer's disease?

There has tremendous progress in recent years in elucidating the mechanisms involved in the deposition of amyloid plaques and the formation of neurofibrillary tangles, and the mechanisms by which plaques and tangles lead to loss of synapses, depletion of neurotransmitters and loss of neurons. As a result, there are many promising strategies being developed to interrupt the destructive processes. For example, research demonstrating the role of oxidative stress in the development of Alzheimer's disease led to the antioxidant trials; vitamin E is now widely used to slow the clinical progression of the disease. The benefits of vitamin E are modest. But many other strategies are under active investigation. Estrogen and anti-inflammatory drugs are being tested both as preventive measures and as treatments for the disease. It has even been suggested that the cholinesterase inhibitors, including donepezil and tacrine, may have some ability to delay the progression of the disease, but this speculation has not been rigorously tested.

If a drug is developed to slow the progression of Alzheimer's disease, when should treatment begin?

Modest advances have been made in identifying treatments that slow the course of Alzheimer's disease. Hence, the question of when should therapy begin is quite relevant. Presumably, the earlier that such treatment is begun, the better the prognosis. But early treatment depends on advances in the science of Alzheimer's disease diagnosis. Currently, a diagnosis of Alzheimer's disease is only made when patients have clear symptoms in at least two cognitive domains, and there is documentation of the progression of their illness. Using this standard guideline, by the time a diagnosis of probable Alzheimer's disease is made, abnormalities in the brain are quite extensive, and have been present for years.

ALZHEIMER'S DISEASE

For optimal disease-modifying treatment, a test is needed to allow accurate diagnosis before symptoms are apparent. To date, no such diagnostic test exists, although this is a very active area of investigation. The likelihood that medication will fully arrest the course of this disease will improve when we can identify the disease at its very earliest stage.

Chapter 4 includes mention of three treatment strategies that may reduce the risk of developing Alzheimer's disease: antioxidants, anti-inflammatory drugs and estrogen. The same three strategies are being pursued as treatments of established Alzheimer's disease. Two other approaches, neurotrophic therapy, and anti-amyloid therapy, are also promising avenues of investigation.

What is the theory behind the use of antioxidants to treat Alzheimer's disease?

The use of antioxidants in the treatment of Alzheimer's disease is based on the "Free Radical Theory of Aging." According to this idea, many manifestations of age-related functional decline and disease are caused by an excess of free radicals in various tissues. Free radicals are highly reactive molecules with unpaired electrons; these unstable molecules will react with many other molecules, often causing damage. Thus, when free radicals are generated in the vicinity of cell membranes, they may cause damage to the lipid and protein components of the membranes. Similarly, free radicals can damage nucleic acids, including DNA.

Free radicals are normally produced by most cells in the body; they are a byproduct of normal cellular metabolism. They serve important functions; for example, free radicals released by inflammatory cells help fight invading bacteria. To prevent free radical damage to normal cells and tissues, the body utilizes a variety of defense mechanisms to neutralize these molecules. Antioxidant enzymes and vitamins are among these defenses.

The "Free Radical Theory of Aging" states that as an individual ages, there is a relative excess of free radicals in relation to defense mechanisms. The result is damage to various organs. For example, free radicals accumulating in the eye may contribute to the development of cataracts; free radicals in blood vessels may contribute to atherosclerotic plaques.

There is some evidence that free radical-mediated damage contributes to the damage to brain tissue found in Alzheimer's disease. Laboratory experiments suggest that the accumulation of amyloid peptides (the major constituents of amyloid plaques in the Alzheimer's disease brain, see Chapter 4) may induce free radical generation in the brain. Whether this process is a major factor in disease progression has not been resolved.

The interest in these mechanisms has been a boon to the vitamin and health food supplement industry. Many products sold over-the-counter claim to have anti-oxidant properties, and are promoted as anti-aging, or cognitive enhancing agents. By and large, experts consider such claims to be without merit. In any case, there is little regulation of such products, and they may cause adverse effects.

Still, there is valid scientific evidence linking free radical damage to Alzheimer's disease. As a result, there have been some controlled clinical trials of anti-oxidant drugs for the treatment of Alzheimer's disease.

One recent large multicenter clinical trial investigated the efficacy of vitamin E, along with another medication with antioxidant properties called selegeline, in slowing the rate of progression of Alzheimer's disease. The results were encouraging. Subjects treated with either vitamin E or selegeline seemed to have a slower rate of disease progression than did subjects treated with placebo. Some experts have expressed caution in interpreting these results, because it is a single study, only moderately demented patients were enrolled, and a similar decline on cognitive tests occurred in subjects treated with antioxidants and placebo.

A controlled trial of a specific formulation of ginkgo biloba has also been reported in the medical literature. A very small cognitive benefit seemed to be associated with the use of ginkgo, compared to a placebo. However, there have been some methodologic criticisms of this study. Further, ginkgo preparations found in health food stores may be quite different from the formulation used in the study.

What is the theory behind the studies of anti-inflammatory treatments for Alzheimer's disease?

In Chapter 4, we noted that in addition to amyloid plaques and neurofibrillary tangles, other alterations have been demonstrated in the Alzheimer's disease brain. Notably, many components of the inflammatory response have been demonstrated.

ALZHEIMER'S DISEASE

Is Alzheimer's disease an inflammatory disease?

There are a number of diseases considered to be inflammatory diseases, that is, the manifestations of the disease are attributed to an inflammatory response that has become destructive rather than protective. Rheumatoid arthritis is an example. In this chronic disease, the body's immune and inflammatory systems attack joint tissue, causing the cardinal features of inflammation: swelling, heat, redness and loss of function.

Patients with Alzheimer's disease do not show the typical signs and symptoms associated with inflammation. They do not have swelling, redness, heat and pain. But they do show subtle laboratory evidence of inflammation. Blood studies demonstrate changes associated with inflammation and altered immune function that may be a reflection of inflammatory activity in the brain.

The key question is whether the inflammation is contributing to the damage to brain cells, or is just an "epiphenomenon," a reaction to the plaques and tangles that does not actually do any harm. This issue has not been resolved.

But there are reasons that many investigators are optimistic that suppressing the brain inflammation with drugs will provide important benefits with regard to Alzheimer's disease.

It appears that patients with rheumatoid arthritis have a reduced risk of Alzheimer's disease; this could be due to a protective effect of the anti-inflammatory drugs used to treat the arthritis. Indeed, many epidemiological surveys suggest that people who take anti-inflammatory drugs have some degree of protection against the disease.

But this type of evidence is not conclusive. Epidemiologic studies can be skewed by many factors, clouding the interpretation of the data. For example, a study showing that patients with Alzheimer's disease are less likely to report past use of prescription anti-inflammatory drugs than a control group of similar age does not prove that such drugs protect against the disease. The patient group may not recall prior drug use due to cognitive deficits, or may have more limited access to physicians likely to prescribe such treatments.

Still, an impressive number of studies report findings suggestive of a protective effect of anti-inflammatory treatment. Along with the laboratory studies showing potentially destructive inflammation in the Alzheimer's disease brain, these studies support efforts to rigorously test whether anti-inflammatory drugs protect against the disease, or slow its progression.

If the inflammatory theory is true, will any anti-inflammatory drug work?

It is not yet known whether any anti-inflammatory drugs are actually beneficial in Alzheimer's disease. If the theory is correct, it is likely that some anti-inflammatory drugs are beneficial while others are not.

There are a large number of anti-inflammatory and immunosuppressive agents that are used to treat various inflammatory/autoimmune diseases. Each disease responds to certain drugs, but not to others. The reason for this variable response is that different inflammatory conditions are caused by different mechanisms (different types of inflammatory cells, and different chemical mediators of inflammation). Each drug is active against some, but not all, inflammatory mechanisms.

In Alzheimer's disease, it is not clear which inflammatory mechanisms contribute to brain cell damage. Some investigators are studying drugs which are effective against complement proteins (an important class of inflammatory mediators apparently involved in Alzheimer's disease). Others are testing drugs which target activated microglial cells, which apparently are the key inflammatory cells in the Alzheimer's disease brain.

Only randomized, controlled clinical trials can determine whether a specific anti-inflammatory treatment strategy is effective.

Which anti-inflammatory drugs show the greatest promise?

At the present time, the class of anti-inflammatory drug that has generated the most excitement is the non-steroidal anti-inflammatory drugs, known as NSAIDs. These are the most widely used anti-inflammatory drugs, and the epidemiologic studies suggest that they may be beneficial in Alzheimer's disease.

The mechanism by which these drugs exert their effects is by inhibiting an inflammatory enzyme called cyclooxygenase, or COX. The activity of COX results in the formation of inflammatory lipid mediators called prostaglandins. NSAIDs are COX inhibitors; they work by reducing the production of prostaglandins in cells. The recent discovery that the two forms of COX (called COX-1 and COX-2) are both present in brain cells provides further evidence that NSAIDs may be useful in treating brain inflammation.

A new class of NSAID, called selective COX-2 inhibitors because they are much more effective at inhibiting COX-2 than COX-1, have been developed and will soon be approved for use in the United States. To a major extent, the anti-inflammatory benefits of NSAIDs result from inhibition of COX-2, while the side effects (such as gastrointestinal bleeding) are caused by inhibition of COX-1. The new selective COX-2 inhibitors are as effective as older NSAIDs in the treatment of inflammation, but they have much less toxicity. Because a number of laboratory studies suggest that COX-2 may contribute to brain cell damage in Alzheimer's disease, there is particular interest in testing the new COX-2 inhibitors in this disease.

What is the status of anti-inflammatory drug trials?

One trial of the synthetic steroid anti-inflammatory drug prednisone has recently been completed; the results are now being analyzed. Several large trials of COX-2 inhibitors are under way. A couple of other types of anti-inflammatory drugs (for example, the antimalarial compound hydroxychloroquine) are now being studied as well.

Since so much is written about anti-inflammatory and antioxidant agents, should everyone take ibuprofen and vitamins to prevent Alzheimer's disease?

NSAIDs such as ibuprofen and naproxen are in widespread use for a variety of symptoms and diseases, and are available without prescription. But there are several reasons why it is not recommended at this time that these drugs be taken to prevent Alzheimer's disease. The theory that anti-inflammatory drugs may be useful in this way has not been proven. While low doses of these drugs are usually well tolerated, it takes higher "prescription" doses to provide significant anti-inflammatory effect, and such doses may cause dangerous side effects.

Many people take antioxidants such as vitamin E in the hope that they may delay Alzheimer's disease or alter its progression. These are relatively benign drugs, but can sometimes cause problems; for example, it has been reported that use of vitamin E can increase the risk of bleeding in individuals taking anticoagulant medication.

As a general rule, all decisions regarding the chronic use of over-the-counter medications and vitamins should be made in consultation with a physician.

What is the evidence that estrogen will be useful in the treatment of Alzheimer's disease?

Apart from its known effects on the female reproductive tract, the cardiovascular system and bone, estrogen has been shown to have important effects on brain cells. There is some evidence that estrogen promotes the survival of brain cells, and that estrogen treatment may provide modest cognitive benefits. As with NSAIDs, epidemiologic surveys indicate that prior use of estrogen may protect against the development of Alzheimer's disease.

Based on these considerations, large scale controlled trials of estrogen have been initiated to determine whether treatment with the hormone can delay the onset of Alzheimer's disease in women, or provide symptomatic benefit to women with the disease. Until the results of such trials are known, the benefits of estrogen treatment with regard to Alzheimer's disease remain unproven. For the present, the decision of a woman and her physician regarding use of estrogen should be based on the known benefits and risks associated with the hormone.

Is there any medication that can prevent the deposition of amyloid in the brain?

Many investigators believe that amyloid peptide, the primary component of amyloid plaques in the Alzheimer's disease brain, is the central etiologic factor in the development of Alzheimer's disease. The discovery of a drug which blocks the formation and/or deposition of amyloid peptide in the brain would be tremendously exciting. The development of such a drug may not be far off.

The successful creation of transgenic mouse models of amyloid deposition in brain represents a major step toward the development of an anti-amyloid drug. The mice were created by inserting mutated human amyloid precursor protein genes (from patients with familial Alzheimer's disease) into the genetic material of mouse cells. The transgenic mice develop amyloid plaques quite similar to those that occur in Alzheimer's disease. They are now being use to screen drugs for a beneficial effect on brain amyloid deposition. There is optimism that an effective anti-amyloid drug will be identified in this manner.

What other strategies are being pursued to slow the course of Alzheimer's disease?

Academic centers and pharmaceutical companies around the world are seeking effective treatments for Alzheimer's disease. Many are working on the types of drugs mentioned above: antioxidant and anti-inflammatory drugs, hormonal treatments and anti-amyloid compounds. A number of other strategies are also being pursued.

One promising example is the search for effective neurotrophic therapy. Neurotrophins are chemicals that support the survival of nerve cells. It is known that one such chemical, called nerve growth factor, is important for the survival of cholinergic brain cells. If levels of nerve growth factor can be increased in areas of brain effected by Alzheimer's disease, progression of the disease may be slowed.

Nerve growth factor cannot be administered by mouth, or by peripheral injection; such modes of treatment do not deliver the compound to the brain. Early attempts to inject nerve growth factor directly into the cerebrospinal fluid (the fluid surrounding the brain) have also not been very successful. However, several compounds that can be administered orally to cause an increased release of nerve growth factor, or increase its effect, in susceptible areas of brain are under development

If a drug is developed that can slow the course of Alzheimer's disease, will symptomatic treatment still be necessary?

In the ideal situation, an inexpensive harmless drug or vitamin could be administered to everyone to reliably prevent Alzheimer's disease, and to eliminate the disease in those already affected. But no drug or supplement is free of risk, and a totally effective treatment is not likely to be found soon. More likely, drugs will be developed that are partially effective in preventing and/or slowing the disease, and individuals will have to balance the potential benefits of such treatment against the risk of side effects and the expense.

The development of universally beneficial treatment is also complicated by difficulties in predicting and diagnosing the disease. While risk may be roughly estimated, no test accurately predicts the development of Alzheimer's disease (except in the rare familial cases). Further, as noted in Chapter 6, diagnosis of established disease is imperfect. So the uncertainty of drug effect is compounded by uncertainty in the identification of individuals to be treated.

Most experts believe that in the near future, the treatment of Alzheimer's disease will involve combinations of drugs. Each individual may require a regimen that includes a symptomatic agent to boost cognition, along with a drug to slow the progression of the disease. Some patients may also require medications to treat behavioral manifestations.

How do we avoid quackery?

Whenever a condition adversely effects millions of people, particularly when the condition causes feelings of desperation, quacks emerge to sell worthless treatments and cures. There are many quacks profiting from the suffering caused by Alzheimer's disease. Typically, these people recount anecdotes of miraculous benefits such as cure of Alzheimer's disease or reversal of the aging process. Most of the time quackery just costs money (it is a billion dollar industry), but sometimes quack remedies can be harmful.

The best way to avoid quackery is to rely on information provided by reputable sources. It is never a good idea to take recommendations from a person or group seeking financial gain from the sale of products. Advertisements should be viewed with skepticism. Reliable advice can be obtained from knowledgeable physicians and from non-profit groups such as the Alzheimer's Association.

ALZHEIMER'S DISEASE

CHAPTER 10

TREATING THE BEHAVIORAL SYMPTOMS

How can the non-cognitive symptoms of Alzheimer's disease be treated?

Management of non-cognitive (i.e. behavioral) symptoms is perhaps the most important challenge facing caregivers and health care professionals. As described in Chapter 7, non-pharmacological management on the part of the caregiver may be quite sufficient. However, when behavioral symptoms become disruptive, emotionally draining, or even physically threatening, medication may be required.

A change in behavior should first prompt a careful investigation into possible environmental or physical precipitating factors. In a patient with cognitive impairment, any physical discomfort may manifest itself as nonspecific agitation. So if an Alzheimer's disease patient suddenly becomes agitated, it is important to look carefully for evidence of common physical discomforts: constipation, urinary tract infection, pneumonia, skin infection, unsuspected bone fracture.

Environmental factors that may trigger agitation include: change in location, change in caregiver, decreased sensory input (whether from insufficient lighting, or decrease in vision or hearing). Figure 10.1 lists some precipitants of abrupt change in behavior patterns of the Alzheimer's disease patient. It is important to note that during the course of the illness behavioral symptoms can wax and wane as well.

The primary approach to the treatment of behavioral symptoms should be

---

CAUSES OF ABRUPT BEHAVIORAL CHANGES

◆ Changes in the environment   ◆ Changes in who is providing care

◆ New medical conditions   ◆ New medications

Figure 10.1 *Lists common reasons for abrupt changes in the behavior of an individual with Alzheimer's disease.*

techniques such as avoidance of precipitating circumstances, distraction and emotional support. The best remedy is often gentle reassurance from a compassionate caregiver.

A host of drugs are available to treat the most difficult behavioral consequences of Alzheimer's disease, such as agitation, sleeplessness, and paranoia. These drugs range from agents with mild sedating properties to antipsychotic drugs. All can be effective at treating behavioral symptoms, though they have markedly different mechanisms of action and potential side effects. Often it is a trial and error process that leads the physician to find a drug that is most effective in diminishing the patient's behavioral symptoms without intolerable adverse effects.

What is the role of antipsychotic medication in Alzheimer's disease?

The class of drugs traditionally used to treat behavioral disturbance in Alzheimer's disease is the neuroleptics (or antipsychotics). These drugs are used to treat psychotic manifestations (e.g. hallucinations, delusions) of psychiatric diseases such as schizophrenia. Thus it is not surprising that these drugs are most useful in Alzheimer's disease when psychotic symptoms are present. But these drugs can also reduce nonspecific agitation and aggressive behavior.

Hallucinations may occur as a result of sensory impairment in a demented individual. If visual hallucinations occur in an Alzheimer's disease patient with visual loss from cataracts, the hallucinations may respond better to cataract extraction than to antipsychotic medication. Similarly, auditory hallucinations can sometimes be treated with hearing aides.

Symptoms that seem to suggest psychotic thinking may be readily attributable to cognitive impairment. For example, an Alzheimer's disease patient who has misplaced an object may fear or believe that it has been stolen. In the later stage of the illness, a patient who does not recognize his or her spouse may believe that there is an intruder in the house. In such circumstances, antipsychotic medication may not be appropriate; gentle reassurance is often effective.

Neuroleptics are often subdivided into high-potency, mid-potency and low-potency drugs. The antipsychotic effect of the drugs is attributed to their dopamine-blocking action, but they also have anticholinergic properties (see section on neurotransmitters in Chapter 3). In general, the lower the potency of a neuroleptic agent, the greater its anticholinergic activity. Because an anticholinergic drug effect will worsen confusion, or even cause delirium, in an Alzheimer's disease patient, high potency neuroleptics are usually prescribed in this setting. Haloperidol is the most common choice.

Unfortunately, because haloperidol has minimal anticholinergic activity, it is prone to cause extra-pyramidal toxicity (i.e. drug-induced Parkinsonism; see Chapter 1). It must be used with great caution in Alzheimer's disease, and should be avoided if any extra-pyramidal features are present (as with the Lewy-Body variant).

When a neuroleptic medication is prescribed to a patient with Alzheimer's disease, the general principals of geriatric pharmacology are particularly important: start with a low dose (in the case of haloperidol, 0.25 or 0.5mg daily), increase slowly if necessary, and repeatedly weigh the benefits against any adverse effects. The effect of neuroleptic medication on a patient with Alzheimer's disease is unpredictable; behavior may get better or worse, and oversedation and increased confusion may occur. Toxic effects, particularly Parkinsonian symptoms such as stiffness, shuffling, tremor and drooling, can occur at any dose.

When neuroleptic drugs are prescribed to patients with schizophrenia, anti-Parkinsonian drugs such as benztropine and amantadine are commonly prescribed as well to treat or prevent the Parkinsonian side effects. These drugs are usually poorly tolerated in patients with Alzheimer's disease; they cause cognitive deterioration, hallucinations or even delirium. These anti-Parkinsonian drugs should never be prescribed prophylactically to patients with Alzheimer's disease. When Parkinsonian side effects complicate the use of neuroleptic medication, the dose of the drug should be reduced, or an alternative treatment substituted.

Are there advantages to new, recently developed antipsychotic medications?

Risperidone is a relatively new antipsychotic medication that seems to cause less Parkinsonism than the older neuroleptics. Early reports suggest that it may be useful in the treatment of delusions and agitation in Alzheimer's disease, but more experience with the drug is needed. Some clinicians have reported that risperidone is less affective than haloperidol in this setting.

Olanzapine is another new antipsychotic medication that is being prescribed to patients with Alzheimer's disease. Olanzapine is related to an earlier drug, clozapine, developed for the treatment of psychotic symptoms refractory to traditional antipsychotic medications; the use of clozapine was limited by its potential to cause serious hematologic toxicity. Olanzapine offers the benefits of clozapine with reduced toxicity. This drug causes much less extra-pyramidal toxicity than drugs such as haloperidol. More experience is needed to determine its efficacy in the treatment of behavioral problems in Alzheimer's disease.

What are the alternatives to antipsychotic medications in the treatment of behavioral disturbances in Alzheimer's disease?

Because of the variable response and risk of toxicity with neuroleptics, alternative drugs to treat agitation in Alzheimer's disease have been actively sought.

Trazodone is a weak antidepressant that is increasingly prescribed to treat agitation in Alzheimer's disease. Anecdotal reports suggest that a majority of patients respond favorably to the drug. Side effects that may occur include orthostatic hypotension (drop in blood pressure with standing), and swelling of the legs. Trazodone is generally considered to be safer than neuroleptic drugs such as haloperidol because it does not cause Parkinsonian symptoms and has no anticholinergic effect.

Two drugs primarily used to treat seizure disorders have also been found to be useful in controlling behavioral symptoms in Alzheimer's disease: carbamazepine and valproic acid. Preliminary studies suggest that both may be effective. These drugs can have toxic effects on the liver and blood cells, so monitoring, including measurement of blood levels, is necessary. Newer anti-epileptic drugs, such as gabapentin, are also being tested for behavioral treatment of Alzheimer's disease.

Are there special considerations in the treatment of depression in patients with Alzheimer's disease?

When drug treatment for depressed mood is considered, the prescribing physician must carefully consider the selection of medication. Any psychotropic drugs may have adverse effects on a patient with dementia, but he risks are much greater with drugs with anticholinergic effects (see Chapter 1). Perhaps the most effective anti-depressant drugs are the tricyclic antidepressants. Within this class, some agents have relatively little anticholinergic activity (e.g. nortriptyline and desipramine), while others have significant anticholinergic effects (e.g. amitriptyline, a drug which should not be prescribed to patients with Alzheimer's disease).

Newer antidepressants, such as the selective serotonin reuptake inhibitors (SSRIs) fluoxetine, paroxetine and sertraline, and the mixed reuptake inhibitor venlafaxine, seem to have a good safety profile in elderly patients with dementia.

Can sedatives be used safely?

There are no sedative medications that are completely safe for use in patients with Alzheimer's disease. Any sedative can worsen cognitive function and impair coordination, increasing the risk of falling. Nonetheless, sometimes sedative medications must be tried to relieve severe agitation and allow sleep.

Benzodiazepines are the most commonly prescribed sedative/hypnotics. Short-acting drugs in this class (lorazepam is an example) are preferred, so if there are adverse effects, they will not last long. Chloral hydrate is a non-benzodiazepine sedative that is often prescribed for Alzheimer's patients. As with all psychotropic medications, it is essential to start at a very low dose, with cautious increases if necessary.

What is the story with melatonin?

Melatonin is a hormone secreted during the night by a tiny gland called the pineal, located adjacent to the brain. Melatonin may play a role in the regulation of the sleep/wake cycle, and there is some evidence that administration of melatonin at night may improve sleep.

Insomnia is very common in elderly people, and levels of melatonin decrease with age. Patients with Alzheimer's disease often have sleep disorders, and it is hoped that melatonin may be useful in restoring normal sleep and reducing nocturnal agitation. Controlled studies have been initiated. At the present time, the efficacy and safety of melatonin have not been established, and so its use cannot recommended. The purity and potency of melatonin preparations available over-the-counter in health food stores and pharmacies is variable.

CHAPTER 11

MEDICAL CARE OF THE PATIENT WITH ALZHEIMER'S DISEASE

Can other medical problems influence the course of Alzheimer's disease?

The typical course of Alzheimer's disease is one of slow deterioration. But it is not uncommon for patients to suffer sudden setbacks, with rapid worsening of cognitive or behavioral symptoms. In many cases, an episode of sudden decline indicates an acute physical or medical problem.

In general, most acute medical conditions present with fairly specific manifestations. But in a patient with Alzheimer's disease, medical problems may be difficult to identify. Typical signs and symptoms may be absent. In fact, the primary manifestation of medical illness in the setting of Alzheimer's disease may be sudden cognitive or behavioral deterioration. The entire range of medical conditions, from constipation or urinary tract infection to ischemic heart disease or cancer can present as non-specific decline in a patient with Alzheimer's disease. In fact, anything causing discomfort can cause apparent global decline. The medical term for this situation is delirium.

It is important that a thorough medical evaluation be conducted when an Alzheimer's patient seems to suffer an accelerated decline.

How can delirium be identified?

Delirium is a state of generalized brain dysfunction caused by an acute medical or physical problem. It is particularly common in patients with an underlying chronic brain disorder such as Alzheimer's disease. Most, if not all, patients with Alzheimer's disease suffer repeated bouts of delirium during the course of their illness, so it is important that caregivers, families and physicians be familiar with the characteristic features of delirium.

Confusion and agitation are common features of both dementia and delirium. But several features usually allow delirium to be identified even when it occurs in the setting of dementia. An individual suffering from delirium usually has an altered, fluctuating level of alertness, while alertness is typically normal in dementia. In contrast to the slow, generally imperceptible decline characteristic of the dementia of Alzheimer's disease, cognitive function and behavior decline noticeably over a period of days to weeks, with marked fluctuations within each day, in an individual suffering from delirium. Hallucinations are more common in delirium than in dementia.

Delirium is a serious, even potentially life-threatening condition. When features of delirium are identified, the treating physician must be notified so that an evaluation can be initiated.

Are there particular concerns regarding the use of medications to treat other illnesses in a patient with Alzheimer's disease?

Any medication, even seemingly innocuous over-the-counter preparations, can cause side effects. While most adverse drug effects are mild and self-limited, most medications carry a risk of serious or fatal toxicity. Every person should be aware of both the benefits and risks of any medication to be taken, so that an informed decision regarding use can be made.

Careful weighing of risks versus benefits of medications is particularly important in older individuals. Aging is associated with many physiologic changes (such as altered absorption, tissue distribution, metabolism and excretion) that lead to variability and unpredictability of drug responses. Older people often take multiple medications, adding the risk of adverse drug interactions. Impairments of hearing and vision increase the risk that medications will be taken improperly, further increasing the risk that a toxic reaction will occur. Based on these considerations, one of the most important principles of geriatric medicine is that medications should be used with great caution in older people, minimizing the number of drugs and the doses. When possible, non-pharmacologic treatments (e.g. dietary changes, exercise, physical therapy) should be substituted for medications.

While the risk of drug toxicity is considerable for any older individual, the risk is still greater for Alzheimer's disease patients. The cognitive deficits increase the risk of compliance errors. At least as important, the brain disease increases the risk of medication-induced delirium.

Almost any medication taken by mouth or by injection can cause delirium in a susceptible individual, but certain drugs carry a particularly high risk. Medications with anticholinergic effects (see Chapter 3) have the greatest risk of inducing delirium. Drugs which cross into the brain are also particularly hazardous. When selecting a specific drug to treat a medical condition, physicians must consider these factors to minimize the risk of delirium.

ALZHEIMER'S DISEASE

CHAPTER 12

LEGAL PLANNING FOR THE ALZHEIMER'S PATIENT

Jay J. Sangerman

When a loved one is faced with the early stages of Alzheimer's disease, given the nature of the illness, practical considerations are often not the first concern. Addressing issues such as healthcare planning and effective property management early can make dealing with the later stages of Alzheimer's easier. This chapter is intended to give an overview of the most important legal issues facing Alzheimer's patients, their loved ones and their physicians. The chapter is divided into three sections: The first section, Planning with the Alzheimer's Patient, discusses how a patient with sufficient decision-making capacity can plan for his/her future property management. This section also discusses how an Alzheimer's patient with sufficient decision-making capacity can specify his/her preferences regarding future healthcare decisions. The second section, Planning in the Later Stages of Alzheimer's, will look at how a patient who no longer possesses sufficient mental capacity for decision-making can be provided for by means of a guardianship proceeding. Paying for Long- Term Care, the third section, discusses various methods for paying for the long-term care necessitated by Alzheimer's disease.

I. PLANNING WITH THE ALZHEIMER'S PATIENT

At the earliest possible time, the Alzheimer's patient and/or the patient's family should consult with his/her attorney for purposes of legal planning for property management, estate planning and advanced directives for medical decision-making. Consideration in such planning should involve the patient's financial security, a determination of who will manage property, the preservation of assets for others, if so desired, and the determination of future medical care. By undertaking proper planning when the Alzheimer's patient has sufficient mental capacity for decision-making, the Alzheimer's patient will be able to impose his/her preferences upon future decision-making for his/her management of property and healthcare. Most important, the legal aspects of planning for the Alzheimer's patient can often be best achieved when there is team effort among the medical and social work providers, the attorney, accountant and financial planner.

PROPERTY MANAGEMENT
What is property management?

For purposes of this chapter, we define property management as the development of a plan whereby there is an efficient and effective system for the administration of property. Under this definition, we are distinguishing "property management" from "financial management." In property management, as defined here, the consideration is "who is going to manage the property," whereas the consideration in financial management is "how is the property going to be invested." Property management necessitates the creation of certain legal documents. A person with sufficient mental capacity can select a family member, a professional (such as an attorney or accountant) or a corporate fiduciary (such as a bank or other financial institution) to manage his/her property.

What is the goal of future planning for property management for the Alzheimer's patient?

The goal of future planning for property management is to seize the opportunity while the Alzheimer's patient has the requisite mental capacity to put into place a mechanism, together with the appropriate documentation, by which the Alzheimer's patient can determine by whom his property will be managed (and spent) if s/he becomes mentally incapacitated. By establishing such a plan, the individual can make determinations for his/her future. In the absence of such a plan, there will likely be the need for a judicial determination of who will manage his/her affairs.

What are the legal devices for the management of another's property?

The legal devices for property management in the hands of another are durable powers-of-attorney, trust agreements and jointly held accounts.

POWER-OF-ATTORNEY
What is a power-of-attorney?

A power-of-attorney is a written instrument by which an individual (the "principal") appoints another as agent to act on his behalf (the "attorney-in-fact"). Generally, a power-of-attorney is limited to property management. In some states, however, the power-of-attorney includes the authority for both property management and medical decision-making.

What mental capacity is required to execute a power-of-attorney?

To execute a valid power-of-attorney, the principal must have the requisite capacity to understand the nature and consequences of his/her executing a document which permits another to act on his/her behalf. Without the requisite mental capacity, an individual cannot legally execute a valid power-of-attorney. Notaries (including health care institutions providing notaries) must be reasonably careful that they do not preside at the execution of a power-of-attorney where the principal lacks the requisite mental capacity to execute a power-of-attorney. If there is a question as to the principal's mental capacity, witnesses should be present to confirm that the principal has capacity and to note their impressions in a written statement that the principal had such capacity. In some instances, legal counsel may advise the use of a video recording to protect the validity of the power-of-attorney. It is also advisable to have a doctor's letter stating that at the time the Alzheimer's patient executed the power-of-attorney, that he had the mental capacity to understand that document he signed.

Does a person with Alzheimer's disease have the requisite mental capacity to execute a power-of-attorney?

A diagnosis of probable Alzheimer's disease is not a sine quo non of incapacity to make fundamental decisions for future planning, nor is it a sine quo non of incapacity to validly execute documents.

Who makes the determination of mental capacity?

The determination of mental capacity should be made by the appropriate medical professional in consultation with the attorney who will be present at the execution of the power-of-attorney. Where the validity of the power-of-attorney may be questioned (e.g. by family members, financial institutions or the taxing authorities), it is much safer to have an attorney (especially one acquainted with the Alzheimer's patient) officiate at the execution of the power-of-attorney. Depending upon the circumstances, the attorney may request a letter from the Alzheimer's patient's doctor setting forth that the patient reasonably has, in the opinion of the doctor, the capacity necessary to understand that s/he is selecting a fiduciary and giving the fiduciary the authority to make property management decisions on his/her behalf.

Is a power-of-attorney valid when the principal becomes incapacitated?

An ordinary power-of-attorney becomes void when the principal becomes incapacitated. Therefore, all states have enacted legislation to permit the execution of a durable power-of-attorney, i.e. a power-of-attorney which survives incapacity. Accordingly, care should be taken to be sure that the power-of-attorney states that it is durable. A durable power-of-attorney will include words such as: "This power-of-attorney shall not be affected by the subsequent disability or incompetence of the principal."

Does the principal lose authority to act in his/her own behalf when s/he executes a power-of-attorney?

The execution of a power-of-attorney does not preclude the principal from acting on his/her own behalf. Unless otherwise stated, the principal and the agent have concurrent authority.

Do all states have the same laws regarding powers-of-attorney?

No. It is important to check one's own state laws since state's have varying requirements regarding powers-of-attorney. For instance, some states require witnesses to the execution of the power-of-attorney. Some states have additional requirements when the power-of-attorney is intended for use in real estate, e.g., filing of the power-of-attorney and/or a full description of the real property written in the power-of-attorney. If a person spends significant time in more than one state, it is advisable to have powers-of-attorney in each state in which the person frequents, especially if the person owns real estate in each state.

I do not wish to give authority to my agent presently. Can the power-of-attorney "spring" into validity upon some stated occurrence?

It all depends upon state law. Some states have statutes authorizing the use of "springing powers-of-attorney." A "springing power-of-attorney" is one in which the agent's authority commences only upon the happening of a certain event, such as mental incapacity. If using a springing power-of-attorney, be extremely cautious that it will be accepted upon the stated occurrence. Financial institutions are especially careful to check that the event has occurred. If the power-of-attorney states that it "springs" into effect upon mental incapacity, be sure that it is written in the power-of-attorney the basis for a determination of incapacity and by whom such determination is to be made, including how many people must concur in the determination of incapacity.

This author does not recommend the use of springing powers-of-attorney unless absolutely necessary. It is better to use a trust agreement (as described later) or for the principal not to give the agent possession of the power-of-attorney, but to have it available for the agent from a third party (perhaps the principal's attorney or accountant) or in the principal's home and accessible only upon necessity.

I have executed a power-of-attorney. Can I revoke it?

Powers-of-attorney can be revoked, but often with difficulty. To revoke a power-of-attorney, one should notify the designated agent(s) and all financial institutions in which the principal has assets, informing them that the power-of-attorney has been revoked. Such notification should be in a writing sent by certified mail, return receipt requested. The principal should also notify his/her attorney and other professional advisors, family members and anyone else whom the principal feels would be helpful in protecting the principal should the agent fraudulently use the power-of-attorney. Generally, the agent cannot be held liable for the use of a revoked power-of-attorney until s/he has been duly notified of the revocation.

When else does a power-of-attorney become terminated?

A power-of-attorney is terminated if the instrument states that it is good only for a specified period of time. Further, and most misunderstood, a power-of-attorney is automatically revoked upon the principal's death. A power-of-attorney cannot be legally used after the agent knows that the principal has died. Upon death, it is the executor (personal representative) or estate administrator who controls the management of property and its distribution. Additionally, some states may permit, or require, the revocation of a power-of-attorney upon the court appointment of a guardian, if a guardian is necessary. In other states, absent fraud, the power-of-attorney remains valid, even after the court appointment of a guardian.

Does a power-of-attorney ever become irrevocable?

Yes, when the principal loses the mental capacity to make property management decisions, the power-of-attorney becomes irrevocable. A court in a guardianship proceeding, however, may have the authority to revoke the power-of-attorney, but the power-of-attorney will be an indicia of whom the principal trusts.

How many agents can there be in a power-of-attorney?

Depending upon state law, there can be an unlimited number of agents to a power-of-attorney. However, the principal must be practical. It becomes unwieldy and confusing to have too many agents. Nevertheless, it is prudent to have more than one agent, when available. With multiple agents, who each have the authority to act individually, should an agent predecease the principal or become incapacitated, there still is someone to act on behalf of the principal. However, where there is no agent able to act and the principal lacks capacity, judicial intervention by means of a guardianship proceeding (as described later) will be required.

If there are multiple agents, must they act together or can they have separate and equal authority?

The power-of-attorney will state whether the agents can act "severally" or must act "together." Requiring the agents to act "together" often makes the agents' functioning unwieldy because of the requirement that all agents sign the financial documents. It is, therefore, generally recommended that the agents be permitted to act "severally." Also, some financial institutions will not accept a power-of-attorney which gives two or more agents equal authority to act. Such institutions want to know that they can rely upon only one individual without any potential dispute from another.

In addition to a general power-of-attorney, should the principal have powers-of-attorney at individual financial institutions?

Yes. It affords greater protection to the principal both while she/he has capacity and afterwards when s/he lacks capacity to have specific powers-of-attorney at individual financial institutions. A specific power-of-attorney is for use at designated financial institutions and for specific accounts at such institutions. Individual financial institutions (banks, brokerage houses, Federal Reserve, Internal Revenue Service) generally have their own form of power-of-attorney. Institutions are often wary of powers-of-attorney because of the potential for fraudulent use. Therefore, it is much easier for the agent to use a power-of-attorney at individual institutions where s/he has the institution's power-of-attorney form and the principal has placed the original power-of-attorney into the institution's files when the principal had capacity. At such times, the institution will also have the agent's signature on file or as part of the power-of-attorney form. It is strongly recommended that if one executes a power-of-attorney that she/he execute both a general power-of-attorney and also a specific power-of-attorney at the various institutions which the person uses.

How many original power-of-attorney should the principal execute?

It is a good idea to execute multiple powers-of-attorney. Institutions will require that they be shown an original. Some institutions may require retaining an original. It is appropriate to give original powers-of-attorney to the agent, the principal's attorney and accountant and other appropriate professionals. Some principals, however, for added security do not give the original powers-of-attorney to the agents, but instead tell them where it is located in case of need.

Need the principal keep powers-of-attorney current?

Unless stated in the power-of-attorney, there is no time after which powers-of-attorneys lose their validity. Even though powers-of-attorney may be of unlimited duration, it is prudent that so long as the principal has the requisite mental capacity, s/he executes new powers-of-attorney every few years. In such way, the financial institutions will be less concerned with the possibility that the power-of-attorney has been revoked.

Can the agent take or gift to others the principal's property?

This is one of the major problems with powers-of-attorney. Unfortunately, while powers-of-attorney are a most useful means by which to manage another's property, powers-of-attorney are an opportunity for financial abuse. In most states, a power-of-attorney cannot legally be used to transfer (i.e., gift) the principal's property unless such authority is specifically granted. Nevertheless, financial institutions often do not ask questions and agents are able to gift the principal's assets without specific authorization. On the other hand, in many instances the principal wishes to give the agent gift-giving authority for purposes of estate and tax planning, as well as for Medicaid planning through the divestment of assets. If desired, gift-giving authority can be limited to the federal gift tax exclusion ($10,000 per person) or broadened to permit gifts of all the principal's assets. If the principal wishes to give the agent authority to gift assets, then such authority should be specifically stated in the power-of-attorney. Prior to accepting the authority to make gifts of another's property, the agent should check with his/her tax advisor as to possible estate tax implications to the agent caused by the gift-giving authority in the event that the agent predeceases the principal.

Are standard forms available for powers-of-attorney?

Most states have standard forms for general, durable powers-of-attorney. They are instantly recognizable by financial institutions. This author recommends the use of such standard forms. Where appropriate, the principal can add powers to the standard form power-of-attorney, such as the authority to make gifts. Although power-of-attorney forms can be purchased at retail stores, it is strongly advised that the principal has his/her attorney complete the power-of-attorney form to best assure that it is properly completed.

What problems should be considered prior to executing a power-of-attorney?

Although a power-of-attorney in the proper hands is most useful and appropriate, a power-of-attorney is potentially a very dangerous instrument by which the principal can be wrongfully divested of his/her assets. The agent, even if not authorized, often has the opportunity to transfer (gift) assets to other people, including the agent himself. A power-of-attorney gives a great deal of authority to an individual without any succinct statement of how the funds are to be managed, spent, given away or preserved. The power-of-attorney does not "spell out" the principal's desires for the use of his/her funds; it is only the giving of authority. There are no "rules" as in a trust agreement (described below) indicating the principal's wishes for how to manage the assets. Accordingly, much thought should be put into deciding who can be trusted with the authority given in a power-of-attorney.

TRUST AGREEMENT
What is a "trust?"

A trust is a legal instrument by which an individual appoints a fiduciary and re-registers the assets in the name of the fiduciary of the trust. The components of a trust are a "grantor" (also known as a settlor, donor or trustor) who places the assets into the trust; a "trustee," who is the fiduciary appointed to manage the assets; a "beneficiary," who receives the benefit of the assets during the continuation of the trust; and the "remaindermen," who receive the assets at the termination of the trust (similar to beneficiaries of a last will and testament).

Are there any rules for the operation of the trust?

The rules for the operation of the trust are found in the trust agreement itself, in addition to the state law which the grantor designates to be controlling.

What are some of the provisions which might be included in the trust agreement?

The trust agreement should specify how the trust assets are to be managed, who is to receive assets (and how much) during the continuation of the trust, the powers of the trustee and the identity of remaindermen of the trust assets. The trust agreement can specify that the grantor (and his/her spouse) wishes to be maintained at home with a certain level of care, even if the cost would exhaust the corpus of the trust to the exclusion of the remaindermen. The trust may give the trustee the authority to purchase long-term care insurance for purposes of planning in the event of an illness requiring nursing home care or homecare attendants. The trust may also provide that the trustee is to make gifts to family members in the same pattern as the grantor has in the past, including payment, e.g., of grandchildren's education expenses and birthday and holiday gifts. The trust may even provide for significant transfers of assets out of the trust for purposes of tax, estate or Medicaid planning. The grantor should discuss with his/her professional advisors the various alternative provisions which she/he may wish to include in the trust agreement. The trust agreement is a very personal document and should be carefully tailored to meet the needs and goals of the grantor. The trust agreement itself should state that the trust is to be governed under the laws and regulations of a particular state.

Unlike a power-of-attorney which generally gives the agent concurrent authority with the principal, a trust may be drafted so that a successor trustee to the grantor (if then serving as trustee) has authority to act only after the grantor trustee's incapacity. The trust should have language which provides for a smooth transition from the grantor as trustee to the successor trustee. Similarly, there should be a smooth transition from one trustee to another. For instance, the trust may provide that upon the written statements of two physicians, one of whom is the trustee's attending physician, that the trustee is unable to handle his/her financial affairs, that the successor trustee or trustees take over. Other language may include consultation with certain family members prior to a change in trustees. Depending upon the grantor's mental capacity, she/he may or may not be the initial trustee of the trust. If the grantor/Alzheimer's patient has sufficient capacity, but is not able to be the sole trustee of the trust, she/he might be the co-trustee with a spouse, child, professional or corporate fiduciary.

Can a trust be amended or revoked?

It depends upon the type of trust. A trust can be designed to be either revocable or irrevocable. The revocable trust is generally used for purposes of property management on behalf of the grantor, who is likely to be the sole beneficiary. An irrevocable trust is generally used in Medicaid planning, various forms of estate and gift tax planning and for the establishment of a managed source of funds for minors.

Who can be a trustee?

Depending upon state law, the trustee can be the grantor alone or the grantor in conjunction with another. The trustee can be a relative, friend or professional such as an attorney or accountant. The trustee also can be a corporate fiduciary such as a bank or stock brokerage company. The decision as to whom to select as trustee should be based on the size of the trust assets and whom the grantor feels is best suited to be the trustee.

What mental capacity is required for the formation of a trust?

A trust is a contract between the grantor and the trustee; therefore, the grantor must have the requisite mental capacity to enter into a contract as defined by the laws of the grantor's home state. When an individual lacks the mental capacity to execute a trust agreement, it may be possible to have a judge order the creation of a trust.

If a person has a trust, need she/he also have a last will and testament?

Yes. A trust provides for the ultimate distribution of those assets which are part of the trust. Often, people do not transfer all their assets into the name of the trust. Therefore, unless the remaining assets are payable upon death to a named beneficiary, probate will be required. For this reason, it is important to have will in addition to the trust. The trust and the will must be coordinated to assign responsibility for the distribution of assets and for payment of taxes and final expenses.

What are the disadvantages of a trust?

One of the predominant disadvantages of a trust is the expense associated with setting up and maintaining the trust. A trust, unlike a power-of-attorney, is a complex instrument. An attorney should draft the trust. Also, the trustee may receive compensation for the performance of his/her duties. Additional work for income tax filings may be required. Another disadvantage is that a trust also can be confusing in the beginning. In order for the trust to be appropriately effective, nearly all of the grantor's assets should be re-registered in the name of the trust. The trustee has the fiduciary obligation to manage the assets and to keep accurate records, including accountings, of the trust activities.

What are the advantages of a trust?

The main advantage of a trust is that the grantor can continue to manage his/her assets until such time that the grantor either becomes incapacitated or no longer wishes to manage his/her assets. At such time, there is a smooth transition to the person who is designated to manage the trust assets. The trust provides rules by which the trustee is to manage the trust assets. There are clear fiduciary obligations which the trustee must follow. In addition, there can be certain reporting obligations as to the management of the trust. Further, it is much easier to manage the assets because they are all in the name of the trust and, in contrast to a power-of-attorney, there should be no concern that the authority of the trustee will not be accepted by financial institutions.

Does a trust require the trustee to render an annual accounting?

It depends upon how the trust is drafted. Such considerations must be discussed with the drafting attorney, taking into account the family relationships and the need, or lack thereof, to require reporting mechanisms. However, in some states, the trustee must render an annual accounting in order to be paid commissions, if the trustee is to receive such commissions.

JOINT ACCOUNTS
What are joint accounts?

A joint account is a bank or investment account registered in the name of more than one person as owners of that account. Depending upon the nature of the specific joint account, each person named in the registration may be empowered to manage and remove the assets from such an account.

Can "joint accounts" be used for asset management?

Joint accounts are another way to manage another individual's assets. Either joint holder of an account generally is able to withdraw funds from the account and manage the account. There are exceptions, however, which are discussed below.

How does a joint account affect an estate plan?

The presumption with joint accounts is that there is a right-of-survivorship between the joint tenants. Therefore, assets placed into a joint account "pass" to the surviving joint holder by "operation of law" not withstanding what the decedent's last will and testament states. The consequence is that one could undo an estate plan by the placement of assets into a joint account. Frequently a parent with two or more children places assets into a joint account with the child who lives near the parent, thereby unintentionally undoing the estate plan as set forth in the last will and testament. For this reason, powers-of-attorney or trust agreements for asset management are often preferable to joint accounts for assets management.

How does a joint account affect estate tax planning?

Joint accounts can undo estate tax planning. Under federal tax law, each individual has a unified estate and gift tax credit which allows $650,000 (credit shelter), which increases to $1,000,000 in the year 2006, to pass free of federal estate and gift taxes. In many states there is a much lower threshold for state estate and gift tax. If spouses place all their assets into jointly held accounts, then the credit shelter could be lost resulting in a significant increase in estate and/or gift taxes to the heirs. For instance, spouses with a joint net worth of $1,300,000 will have no federal estate or gift taxes if the assets are evenly split between them and, upon the death of the first-to-die spouse, the assets of the decedent do not "pass" to the surviving spouse. If all the assets are held jointly between the husband and wife, the surviving spouse will die owning all the assets, thereby incurring for the heirs a federal estate tax of $202,505, which could have been fully avoided with proper planning.

What are the advantages of jointly held property?

The advantages of jointly held property are simplicity of asset management and the lack of legal costs for the preparation of documents for such management. Another advantage of jointly held property is that the property generally will "pass" to the surviving joint tenant upon the death of the first-to-die without the need nor cost of probate.

Can either joint tenant withdraw funds from a joint account or manage the property within the joint account?

The answer depends upon the type of account and the institution holding the account. For instance, either joint tenant can generally withdraw funds from a jointly held bank account. However, if the withdrawal of the property would create a loss of interest to the account holders or a penalty, many banks, for their own protection, require the signatures of each joint tenant. With stock certificates, if the stocks are held in certificate form, the signatures of both joint tenants will likely be required by the stock transfer agent; however, if the stocks are held by a stock broker in "street name," i.e. in the name of the financial institution, then only one joint tenant will generally need to sign. Also, with transfers of real estate, both joint tenants generally will have to sign the deed transferring the property.

What is the disadvantage of jointly held assets?

The disadvantage of jointly held accounts is that joint accounts may undo an estate plan by causing certain assets unintentionally to go to certain individuals when they were really intended to pass pursuant to the person's last will and testament. Also, such accounts give an individual the opportunity to remove property from the control of the joint tenant (who placed all the property into the joint accounts) when that may not have been the intent of the person who placed all the funds into the joint account.

A word of caution: Prior to any changes in the distribution or registration of property, it is imperative to seek the advice of an estate planning and tax professional, who may be an accountant, attorney, financial planner or all of the above. Changes in property management can have significant tax consequences.

PLANNING FOR FUTURE MEDICAL DECISION-MAKING
What kind of planning should be done for the Alzheimer's patient in regard to future medical decision-making?

An Alzheimer's patient (and also every other adult) with sufficient capacity to execute an advance directive for medical decision-making should do so at the earliest opportunity. Advance medical directives include either or both (i) the setting forth of one's medical wishes which are to be followed in the event of mental incapacity and/or (ii) the designation of a surrogate to make medical decisions without necessarily any reference to written instructions. In 1990, the United States Supreme Court, in the case of Nancy Cruzan, stated that every American has the fundamental right under the constitution to make his/her own medical decisions. However, the Court went on to state that it is up to each individual state to determine who, if anyone, can make medical decisions for one unable to make his/her own decisions. State laws, therefore, vary on advance medical directives and should be carefully reviewed.

What is a Living Will?

A living will is a document in which one states his/her medical wishes to be followed in the event that s/he cannot communicate his/her wishes at some time in the future. For instance, in a living will, an individual might state that she/he does not wish to be given medical treatment, such as antibiotics or artificial life support, which would only serve to prolong the dying process. All states have laws authorizing the validity of Living Wills.

What problems can be encountered with a Living Will?

A living will is intended to give "instruction" to the provider of medical care. Therefore, it must be carefully drafted so as to avoid ambiguities and to succinctly state the principal's wishes, yet be broad enough to encompass general medical treatment. If one executes a living will, the individual should consider using a "form" document which is readily recognizable to medical providers. Some states provide a recommended form for such use. In other states, where the state legislature has not provided a form, certain well-recognized organizations have forms which are well drafted and easily understood by medical practitioners. Also, certain religious organizations have published their own forms of living wills. If a living will is ambiguous, the medical provider may not be able to discern the patient's wishes and require judicial intervention.

Can an individual appoint an agent to make medical decisions when the individual cannot communicate his/her preferences?

Many, but not all, states have statutes governing the appointment of an agent to make surrogate medical decisions. Such documents may be called a "Health Care Proxy" or "Power of Attorney for Health Care." State laws vary on the form for this advance directive, as well as its use.

Is the appointment of an agent in one state valid in other states?

Such documents are relatively new to the law. Twenty-nine states with statutes relating to advance medical directives expressly permit agents appointed in documents executed in other states to make health care decisions on behalf of incapacitated principals. However, the conditions under which the agent can make medical decisions varies among the states. It is, therefore, recommended that someone with homes in different states have documents executed in the form used in each state in which they frequent.

What mental capacity is required to appoint an agent to make medical decisions?

It is up to state law. Many states have laws which state that everyone is presumed competent to execute an appointment of a healthcare agent. In such instance, the level of requisite mental capacity is far below that required for the execution of a living will.

What considerations should be taken prior to the execution of a living will or appointment of an agent?

There probably can be no more important document executed than an advance medical directive; yet, people often execute them without full deliberation. When possible, prior to execution of an advance medical directive, the principal should consider the moral and religious implications, if any, of executing such a document. If the person is religious, she/he should consult with his/her religious leader. Certainly, prior to the appointment of an agent, when possible, the principal should inform the agent of his/her medical wishes.

Who should be the agent?

Generally in most states anyone can be the agent except for the treating physician. Careful consideration must be given to whether the agent can be "trusted" to give the medical instruction which the principal would want. Such instructions may include the giving, or withholding, of artificial nutrition and hydration and/or the use of a ventilator. A loving spouse, whom the principal fully trusts, may not be the proper agent to make medical decisions pertaining to the withholding of life sustaining treatment.

How many agents can there be?

In most states which have laws on surrogate decision-making, there can be only one agent acting at a time. Therefore, there is generally a primary agent and an alternate agent named in the surrogate document.

Can the agent make any medical decision for the principal?

It depends upon the state. In some states, for instance, artificial nutrition and hydration are considered on a different level than medical treatment. In such states, the agent, if she/he is to have the authority to make decisions pertaining to the provision, or withdrawal, of artificial nutrition and hydration, must have been given the specific authority to make such decisions and know the principal's wishes.

Should a person execute both a living will and a document appointing an agent?

There is a split within the legal community on this issue. Some feel that if the individual has an appropriate person(s) to appoint as agent(s), then it is best to have only the appointment of an agent. Therefore, there is no written document which could be ambiguous as to the principal's wishes. Others within the legal community prefer both so that the living will acts as a guide to the agent and is available as an expression of the principal's wishes in the event the agent is not available. The issue to consider is that the living will limits the authority and flexibility of the agent in that the agent must follow the living will.

Can there be surrogate decision-making in the absence of an advance directive?

It depends upon the law of the particular state. Some states permit "interested" parties to give instructions for the provision of medical care. In such states, the statutes provide for priority of decision-makers. This means that in the absence of an advance directive appointing an agent, state law will determine who, if anyone, has authority for surrogate decision-making. In such matters, the hospital or nursing home risk management or ethics committee may have to intervene and determine who, if anyone, has the authority to express the wishes of the patient.

If an individual has both a power-of-attorney and an advance medical directive, will all decisions be able to be made in the event of incapacity?

Generally, if there is a valid power-of-attorney and an advance medical directive, all relevant decisions will be able to be made for the individual in the event of incapacity.

Is it useful to have a doctor's letter with regard to mental capacity?

Without question, the answer is "yes." Financial institutions are concerned with the validity of powers-of-attorney and the capacity of the Alzheimer's patient at the time of the execution of such a document. Therefore, it is helpful to have a note in the patient's medical file and a contemporaneous letter in the attorney's file stating, if it is the case, that the individual has the capacity to execute a power-of-attorney, a trust agreement and/or an advance medical directive.

II. PLANNING IN THE LATER STAGES OF ALZHEIMER'S DISEASE

At this stage, there are not as many options. In the event that there has been no advance planning by a patient for either property management or healthcare decision-making and the patient no longer possesses sufficient mental capacity to allow for such planning, court intervention becomes necessary. Courts appoint an individual, usually called a guardian, to make decisions; such decisions vary from strictly financial decisions to health or personal or a combination thereof depending upon the powers decided by the judge.

PROPERTY MANAGEMENT AND MEDICAL DECISION MAKING FOR THE INCAPACITATED IN THE ABSENCE OF PROPERTY MANAGEMENT AND MEDICAL DIRECTIVES

How is a guardian appointed?

A guardian is a court appointment made after a judicial finding of incapacity. The guardian may be a family member, a friend or a stranger who never knew the individual. Because the guardian may not have known the ward, the guardian may be unable to ascertain the wishes of the ward. Therefore, unlike where there are directives of property management and medical decision-making indicating the principal's wishes, the court-appointed guardian will likely apply a "best interest" test for decision-making, which could be contrary to that which the individual actually would have wanted. Had the individual performed the proper planning, the individual's choices would have been followed. Every state has its own laws of guardianship.

What powers is the guardian given?

A guardian is given certain powers over the incapacitated person. If there is an advance medical directive, but no mechanism for property management, then the guardian may be given authority only over property management and the designated advance directive agent will continue to make medical decisions. Similarly, if there is a plan for property management, but no medical directive, it is possible that the court will continue the property management plan put into place when the incapacitated individual had capacity and give the guardian authority only over medical decision-making.

Who makes the determination of mental capacity?

Except as otherwise set forth in a state's guardianship statute, only a court can make the legal determination of mental incapacity. Generally, a judge will make such determination after observing the alleged incapacitated individual and hearing testimony from an examining psychiatrist and people familiar with the alleged incapacitated individual. Nevertheless, certain state statutes have provisions for the determination of mental capacity by physicians in specific instances, especially in the case of surrogate medical decision-making. Also, certain legal documents, such as a trust agreement, may set forth how to determine incapacity so as to remove a trustee.

What can medical providers do to protect themselves when treating patients of questionable mental capacity?

There cannot be informed consent without the requisite mental capacity. An unconsented "touch," e.g., a medical procedure without patient permission, can be an assault and battery, subjecting the physician and provider institution to liability. Therefore, unless there is a specific statutory guideline for the determination of mental incapacity, in cases of questionable capacity, medical providers should consider looking to the courts for such a determination prior to undertaking elective medical procedures, including the transferring of patients to other medical institutions. Medical providers should speak with their legal counsel to best protect themselves and, if necessary, to determine how to expedite a judicial determination of capacity. Should the court determine that the patient lacks mental capacity, then the court should determine who shall be the medical and property decision-maker, as well as the authority of the decision maker (i.e. the guardian or special guardian).

Is it safe for medical providers to make determinations of mental capacity for the execution of legal documents?

Unless otherwise authorized by statute, medical providers should restrict their determination of mental capacity for the execution of legal documents to a determination solely based on "professional opinion." It is the court, if necessary, which will make the legal determination.

III. PAYING FOR LONG-TERM CARE

The questions below address concerns involved with financing the long-term care often necessitated by Alzheimer's disease:

Is there insurance available to cover nursing home care?

Long-term care insurance is available, but it generally requires a medical examination to qualify.

If I qualify, what should I look for in long-term insurance?

There are certain policy provisions which should be considered. Among them are:

he 'gatekeepers,' which must be satisfied before the policy will pay for the nursing home care: coverage of Alzheimer's-type dementia; possible requirement for a prior three-day hospital stay; number of ADLs (activities of daily life - feeding, dressing, bathing, toileting and maneuvering) which cannot be performed prior to the policy paying;

the exclusion period prior to payment which should be carefully considered together with Medicare benefits and Medigap benefits;

daily coverage and number of months of coverage;

an inflation rider;

a waiver of premium so that the insured stops paying premiums once s/he is in a nursing home or receiving care at home and the insurance company has started to pay benefits; and

nonforfeiture of benefits so that should the insured stop paying premiums, there might be some return to the insured on the investment.

Do long-term care policies cover care at home?

Some of the policies cover care at home or offer a combination of care plans, such as six years of homecare or three years of nursing home care or any combination thereof.

Where do I receive information about long-term care insurance?

Check with the department of insurance in your state. The department of insurance probably has a book setting forth the various options available within a long-term care insurance policy. Such information booklets may also compare policies and costs of various insurance carriers. Insurance agents should also be able to provide the consumer with an information booklet prepared by the insurance industry. Information can also be obtained from local departments of the aging and senior citizen organizations. Most important, it is wise to contact several companies and agents before purchasing long-term care insurance. Ask the insurance agents for outlines of coverage summarizing the policy's benefits and highlighting important features. Be sure to compare benefits, facilities covered, exclusions and premiums.

Does Medicare pay for nursing home care?

Medicare payments for nursing home care are very limited. At the most, Medicare will pay for 100 days of nursing home care with a deductible from day 21 to day 100.

What are the criteria for Medicare payment for the nursing home stay?

Medicare will pay only if the following criteria are met: that there was a prior three day in-patient hospital stay; that the hospital stay was within 30 days of admission to the nursing home; and that the nursing home stay is for "skilled nursing care" as defined by Medicare. Further, the nursing home stay must be for the same condition as was the prior hospitalization.

When will I know if Medicare will cover my nursing home stay?

The hospital social worker will be able to tell the patient and/or family the probability of whether Medicare will cover the nursing home stay. The final determination, however, will occur only after admission into a nursing home.

Will Medicare pay for homecare?

Medicare will pay for very limited home health services when the patient is under the care of his physician. In order to qualify, one must be in need of intermittent skilled nursing care, physical or speech therapy or occupational therapy. The services must be provided by a home health agency.

Can life insurance be used to pay for long-term care?

Yes. Certain life insurance companies offer "qualified accelerated death benefits." Under recent changes to the Internal Revenue Code section 101(a), these payments are income tax free. This benefit is payable only if the insured becomes terminally ill, i.e. has an illness or physical condition that is reasonably expected to result in death within 12 months of the date on which the accelerated benefit is paid. Under the new and developing law, there is also another living benefit that can be purchased that provides accident and health benefits upon the occurrence of certain morbidity risks. These insurance benefits should be considered as only one of the methods to pay for long-term care; they should not be viewed as a substitute for long-term care insurance. Prior to purchasing such benefits, the insured should speak with his/her tax advisor as this is a new and developing tax law with specific regulations and there are specific conditions that must be met. Also, there are certain possible income tax deductions available for the payment of the premiums for long-term care insurance.

Will Medicaid pay for long-term care in a nursing home?

Yes, but only under certain circumstances. Because the laws governing Medicaid are a combination of state and federal laws, it is important to check one's own state law. In all states, Medicaid will pay for nursing home care, but only when certain specific conditions are met. Laws governing Medicaid can be dramatically different from one state to another and the differences will accelerate as Congress changes federal laws. Medicaid in some states also pays for homecare attendants.

Does the Alzheimer's patient need to be poor to qualify for Medicaid?

Medicaid is a program for the poor. However, for the elderly and the disabled, Medicaid has become the source of payment for healthcare for many. It is possible to divest oneself of assets in order to qualify for Medicaid. However, when one divests oneself, one creates a period of ineligibility during which Medicaid will not pay for nursing home or nursing home-type care. The longest effective period of ineligibility created by divestment of assets is 36 months from the date of divestment, except in the case of an irrevocable trust with income back to the individual, in which case the maximum period of ineligibility is 60 months from the date of transfer, (if divestment is not done appropriately, one could extend the period of ineligibility). The period of ineligibility is counted from date of transfer and not from date of entry into a nursing home.

Can the Alzheimer's patient divest him/herself of assets after admission to a nursing home?

Generally an individual can divest him/herself at any time, even after entry into a nursing home. However, check local law and be careful of the provisions of the nursing home contract. Under federal Medicare laws, a nursing home cannot evict an individual who has exhausted his/her assets for medical care, who is eligible for Medicaid and for whom the only source of payment is Medicaid.

Does one require special advice as to divestment of assets?

Absolutely. Do not undertake a plan of divestment without expert advice. When one divests, s/he creates a period during which Medicaid will not pay for nursing home care. It is, therefore, important to receive advice from one knowledgeable in Medicaid planning prior to any divestment. Prior to any contemplated divestment, there must be an evaluation of the income and estate/gift tax consequences of such contemplated divestment. Also, it is important to inquire of experts as to whom are legally responsible relatives who can be held liable for payments made by Medicaid.

Can an advanced Alzheimer's patient who does not have the capacity to participate in financial decision-making be divested of assets?

The answer depends upon state law. In many states, it is possible to petition a court for permission to transfer assets. This procedure is generally done within a guardianship proceeding.

Where can one go for advice about planning for long-term care?

Family members and/or friends should consult with legal counsel, tax advisors, insurance agents and financial planners; and local social service agencies, hospital social workers, nursing home social workers and departments of the aging in their municipality. Social service agencies, including hospitals and nursing homes generally maintain a listing of resources for guidance in long-term planning for the Alzheimer's patient.

Are there any other sources of payment to the Alzheimer's patient that should be considered?

Yes, a legally disabled individual who is not yet a recipient of Social Security may be eligible to receive Social Security Disability income if s/he worked a sufficient period of time. Social Security Disability payments are based upon the amount of time worked and income earned; the payments are not subject to an income and asset test. There is no age requirement. Also, after one has been on Social Security Disability for two years, she/he qualifies for Medicare medical coverage.

What if the Alzheimer's patient does not qualify for Social Security Disability payments. Are there other sources of funds available?

If one does not qualify for Social Security Disability, then it is possible to qualify for Supplemental Security Income. To qualify, the individual must be disabled or elderly and have assets not greater than $2,000 in addition to a burial fund of not more than $1,500. The maximum allowable income level changes each year. One should also check the availability of food stamps, senior citizen housing allowances or rent reductions and welfare.

CONCLUSION

It is imperative to seize the opportunity at the earliest possible time to plan for the future financial and medical care for the Alzheimer's patient and his/her family. Consult with the professionals in such planning. An excellent place to begin is with the medical providers who should maintain a current list of resources for information and advice. Medical providers who do not have such resource information should, as a service to their patients, obtain such resource information and keep it available for the Alzheimer's patient and his/her caregivers. By proper planning, the quality of care for the Alzheimer's patient and his/her family and significant others can be enhanced, while providing the appropriate security and peace of mind for those caring for the Alzheimer's patient.

ALZHEIMER'S DISEASE

CHAPTER 13

SHOULD WE PARTICIPATE IN RESEARCH STUDIES?

Every patient with Alzheimer's disease, and every relative and friend, seeks to optimize quality of life in the face of this devastating disorder. This is, and should be, the primary goal. Health care professionals, the doctors, nurses, therapists and social workers who provide care to the patients and families, work toward the same goal.

The goal of medical research is distinct: to increase understanding of the illness, and to develop treatments. While the ultimate goal is to optimize quality of life, the immediate goal of researchers conducting studies is to learn about the disease and its treatments.

Much of medical research depends on information obtained from patients with the disease. All treatments must be tested on patients. Without the cooperation of patients and their families, research will not move forward.

Usually, research is a slow process. While participation in research studies always promotes an increase in knowledge of Alzheimer's disease, in most cases the research does not directly benefit the patients who participate. Patients who provide specimens (such as blood or cerebrospinal fluid) do not personally benefit at all. Patients who participate in treatment studies may or may not gain any benefit. In participating, they agree to follow the conditions of the study, and the study is designed to answer questions (e.g. does a certain drug work better than a placebo), rather than to help individual participants.

In considering participation in research, patients and families should understand that the goals of the research and their personal goals are not always identical. They should understand the legal and ethical guidelines of medical research.

So why participate?

Most people decide to participate in research because they wish to help find better treatments, hopefully for themselves, but in any case for future sufferers. Participation in research can be gratifying, adding meaning and satisfaction to the struggle with the disease. While the hope for an immediate cure will be frustrated, the hope to contribute to greater understanding of this disease and to the development of effective treatments in the future will not be frustrated. Participation does have some immediate benefits, primarily the interaction with a group of skillful, compassionate and dedicated research personnel and physicians. Many patients find research participation rewarding, and maintain a long-term relationship with research centers, joining several studies.

CHAPTER 14

WHAT DOES THE FUTURE HOLD?

There are many scientists and clinicians at many institutions around the world working to improve understanding, prevention and treatment of Alzheimer's disease. As a result of these efforts, there have been many advances in recent years. The processes that cause dysfunction of brain cells in this disease are much better understood now, and the genetic factors that contribute to these processes are clearer. Just a few years ago, the first effective treatment, tacrine, became available. Today, most patients with Alzheimer's disease benefit from cholinergic therapy.

It is certain that this progress will continue. The discovery of animal models of the disease, along with the elucidation of genes and proteins that can cause the disease, has led to optimism among investigators that new treatments will be found. Drugs that may slow the deposition of amyloid in brain are in development. The reported success of antioxidant treatment is encouraging, and there is tremendous enthusiasm for the potential benefits of anti-inflammatory drugs. Many trials are in progress, testing drugs that may improve cognitive function, control behavioral symptoms, and slow the rate of disease progression. Preventive treatment strategies are also being studied in controlled clinical trials.

In addition to the search for medications to treat Alzheimer's disease, health care professionals are investigating ways to ease the burden on families. Studies are under way to find methods to ease caregiver stress. New types of specialized care settings are being tested.

Even during periods of widespread cutbacks in governmental spending, few argued for limiting the resources devoted to research in Alzheimer's disease. In the present strong economy, funding for biomedical research in general is growing, including increased spending on basic and clinical research studies on Alzheimer's disease. The efforts will continue, and the outlook is good.

ALZHEIMER'S DISEASE

CHAPTER 15

SELECTED REFERENCES

The volume of literature published on Alzheimer's disease is enormous. The articles and books included here, which support the answers provided in the preceding chapters, represent a tiny fraction of available source material. Of necessity the categories overlap; at times, the assignment of a reference to one category is arbitrary.

Genetics, epidemiology and risk factors

Van Duijn, C.M., Tanja, T.A., Haaxma, R., Schulte, W., Saan, R.J., Lameris, A.J., Antonides-Hendriks, G. and Hofman, A. Head trauma and the risk of Alzheimer's disease. Am J Epidemiol 135:775-782, 1992.

Mendez, M.F., Underwood, K.L., Zander, B.A., Mastri, A.R., Sung, J.H. and Frey, W.H.,II Risk factors in Alzheimer's disease: A clinicopathologic study. Neurology 42:770-775, 1992.

Schellenberg G.D., Bird T.D., Wijsman E.M., Orr H.T., Anderson L., Nemens E., White J.A., Bonnycastle L., Weber J.L., Alonso M.E., Potter H., Heston L.L., Martin G.M. Genetic linkage evidence for a familial Alzheimer's disease locus on chromosome 14. Science 258:668-671, 1992.

Bachman, D.L., Wolf, P.A., Linn, R.T., Knoefel, J.E., Cobb, J.L., Belanger, A.J., White, L.R. and D'Agostino, R.B. Incidence of dementia and probable Alzheimer's disease in a general population: The Framingham Study. Neurology 43:515-519, 1993.

Small, G.W., Leuchter, A.F., Mandelkern, M.A., La Rue, A., Okonek, A., Lufkin, R.B., Jarvik, L.F., Matsuyama, S.S. and Bondareff, W. Clinical, neuroimaging, and environmental risk differences in monozygotic female twins appearing discordant for dementia of the Alzheimer type. Arch Neurol 50:209-219, 1993.

Stern, Y., Gurland, B., Tatemichi, T.K., Tang, M.X., Wilder, D. and Mayeux, R. Influence of education and occupation on the incidence of Alzheimer's disease. J Amer Med Assoc 271:1004-1010, 1994.

ALZHEIMER'S DISEASE

Levy-Lahad E., Wijsman E.M., Nemens E., Anderson L., Goddard K.A.B., Weber J.L., Bird T.D., Schellenberg G.D. A familial Alzheimer's disease locus on chromosome 1. Science 269:970-973, 1995.

McGeer PL, Schulzer M, McGeer EG: Arthritis and anti-inflammatory agents as possible protective factors for Alzheimer's disease: A review of 17 epidemiologic studies. Neurology 47:425-432, 1996.

Cruts M, Hendriks L, Van Broeckhoven C: The presenilin genes: A new gene family involved in Alzheimer disease pathology. Hum Mol Genet 1996. 5:1449-1455, 1996.

Roses AD: Apolipoprotein E alleles as risk factors in Alzheimer's disease. Annu Rev Med 47:387-400, 1996.

Wisniewski T, Dowjat WK, Permanne B, Palha J, Kumar A, Gallo G, Frangione B: Presenilin-1 is associated with Alzheimer's disease amyloid. Am J Pathol 151:601-610, 1997.

Hutton M, Hardy J: The presenilins and Alzheimer's disease. Hum Mol Genet Suppl R:1639-1646, 1997.

Stewart WF, Kawas C, Corrada M, Metter EJ: Risk of Alzheimer's disease and duration of NSAID use. Neurology 48:626-632, 1997.

Evans DA, Hebert LE, Beckett LA, Scherr PA, Albert MS, Chown MJ, Pilgrim DM, Taylor JO: Education and other measures of socioeconomic status and risk of incident Alzheimer disease in a defined population of older persons. Arch Neurol 54:1399-1405, 1997.

Evans DA: The epidemiology of dementia and Alzheimer's disease: An evolving field. J Am Geriatr Soc 44:1482-1483, 1997.

Farlow MR: Alzheimer's disease: Clinical implications of the apolipoprotein E genotype. Neurology Suppl 6:S30-S34, 1997.

Munoz DG: Is exposure to aluminum a risk factor for the development of Alzheimer disease? No. Arch Neurol 55:737-739, 1998.

Growdon JH: Apolipoprotein E and Alzheimer disease. Arch.Neurol. 55:1053-1054, 1998.

Alloul K, Sauriol L, Kennedy W, Laurier C, Tessier G, Novosel S, Contandriopoulos A: Alzheimer's disease: a review of the disease, its epidemiology and economic impact. Arch. Gerontol. Geriatr. 27:189-221, 1998.

Blacker D, Tanzi RE: The genetics of Alzheimer disease -- and future prospects. Arch Neurol 55:294-296, 1998.

De Strooper B, Saftig P, Craessaerts K, Vanderstichele H, Guhde G, Annaert W, Von Figura K, Van Leuven F: Deficiency of presenilin-1 inhibits the normal cleavage of amyloid precursor protein. Nature 391:387-390, 1998.

Duff K: Transgenic models for Alzheimer's disease. Neuropathol Appl Neurobiol 24:101-103, 1998.

Etiology

Drachman, D.A. and Leavitt, J. Human memory and the cholinergic system. Arch Neurol 30:113-121, 1974.

Sapolsky, R.M. and McEwen, B.S. Stress, glucocorticoids and their role in degenerative changes in the aging hippocampus. In: Treatment Development Strategies for Alzheimer's Disease, edited by Crook, T., Bartus, R., Ferris, S. et al., New Canaan: Mark Powley Associates, 1986, p. 151-172.

Sisodia, S.S., Koo, E.H., Beyreuther, K., Unterbeck, A. and Price, D.L. Evidence that beta-amyloid protein in Alzheimer's disease is not derived by normal processing. Science 248:492, 1990.

Kosik, K.S. Alzheimer's disease: A cell biological perspective. Science 256:780-783, 1992.

Arriagada, P.V., Growdon, J.H., Hedley-Whyte, E.T. and Hyman, B.T. Neurofibrillary tangles but not senile plaques parallel duration and severity of Alzheimer's disease. Neurology 42:631-639, 1992.

Caporaso, G.L., Gandy, S.E., Buxbaum, J.D., Ramabhadran, T.V. and Greengard, P. Protein phosphorylation regulates secretion of Alzheimer â/A4 amyloid precursor protein. Proc Natl Acad Sci USA 89:3055-3059, 1992.

Hardy, J.A. and Higgins, G.A. Alzheimer's disease: The amyloid cascade hypothesis. Science 256:184-185, 1992.

Richardson, J.S., Subbarao, K.V. and Ang, L.C. On the possible role of iron-induced free radical peroxidation in neural degeneration in Alzheimer's disease. Ann NY Acad Sci 648:326-327, 1992.

Good, P.F. and Perl, D.P. Aluminum in Alzheimer's. Nature 362:418, 1993.

...heimer Disease. New York: Raven

...rofibrillary tangles initiate plaque
...hat leads to NFT pathology? Neurobiol

...ndrini R, Barbour R, Berthelette P, Blackwell C,
...lson T, Gillepsie F, Guido T, Hagopian S,
...K, Lee M, Leibowitz P, Lieberburg I, Little S,
...ue L, Montoyo Zavala,M., Mucke L, Paganini L,
Penn... ...opment of neuropathology similar to Alzheimer's disease in... ...enic mice overexpressing the 717V-F -amyloid precursor protein. Nature 373:523-527, 1995.

Rogers J, Webster S, Lue LF, Brachova L, Civin WH, Emmerling M, Shivers B, Walker D, McGeer P: Inflammation and Alzheimer's disease pathogenesis. Neurobiol Aging 17:681-686, 1996.

Aguzzi A, Brandner S, Marino S, Steinbach JP: Transgenic and knockout mice in the study of neurodegenerative diseases. J Mol Med 74:111-126, 1996 .

Alonso AD, Grundke-Iqbal I, Iqbal K: Alzheimer's disease hyperphosphorylated tau sequesters normal tau into tangles of filaments and disassembles microtubules. Nature Med 2:783-787, 1996.

Coleman PD, Greenberg BD: Development of animal models of Alzheimer's disease: Status of the field - Editorial. Neurobiol Aging 17:151-151, 1996.

Yankner BA: New clues to Alzheimer's disease: Unraveling the roles of amyloid and tau. Nature Med 2:850-852, 1996.

Beyreuther K, Masters CL: Alzheimer's disease - Tangle disentanglement. Nature 383:476-477, 1996.

Beyreuther K, Masters CL: Alzheimer's disease - The ins and outs of amyloid-beta. Nature 389:677-678, 1997.

Whitehouse PJ: Genesis of Alzheimer's disease. Neurology 48 Suppl 7:S2-S71997.

Markesbery WR: Oxidative stress hypothesis in Alzheimer's disease. Free. Radic. Biol Med 23:134-147, 1997.

Hardy J: The Alzheimer family of diseases: Many etiologies, one pathogenesis? Proc Natl Acad Sci USA 94:2095-2097, 1997.

Hyman BT, Gomez-Isla T: The natural history of Alzheimer neurofibrillary tangles and amyloid deposits. Neurobiol Aging. 18:386-387, 1997.

Lamb BT: Presenilins, amyloid-Beta and Alzheimer's disease. Nature Med. 3:28-29, 1997.

Kosik KS: Presenilin interactions and Alzheimer's disease. Science 279: 463-464, 1998.

Cummings JL, Vinters HV, Cole GM, Khachaturian ZS: Alzheimer's disease - Etiologies, pathophysiology, cognitive reserve, and treatment opportunities. Neurology 51 Suppl 1:S2-S171998

Differential diagnosis and assessment

Folstein, M., Folstein, S. and Mchugh, P. The Mini-Mental State Examination. J Psychiatr Res 12:189-198, 1975.

McKhann, G., Drachman, D., Folstein, M., Katzman, R., Price, D. and Stadlan, E.M. Clinical diagnosis of Alzheimer's disease: Report of the NINCDS-ADRDA Work Group. Neurology 34:939-944, 1984.

Rosen, W.G., Mohs, R.C. and Davis, K.L. A new rating scale for Alzheimer's disease. Am J Psychiatry 141:1356-1364, 1984.

Lipowski, Z.J. Delirium in the elderly patient. N Engl J Med 320: 578-582, 1989.

Lipowski, Z.J. Delirium: acute confusional states, New York: Oxford University Press, 1990. Ed. 2

DeKosky, S.T., Harbaugh, R.E., Schmitt, F.A., Bakay, R.A.E., Chang Chui, H., Knopman, D.S., Reeder, T.M., Shetter, A.G., Senter, H.J., Markesbery, W.R. and Intraventricular Bethanecol Study Group, Cortical biopsy in Alzheimer's disease: Diagnostic accuracy and neurochemical, neuropathological, and cognitive correlations. Ann Neurol 32: 625-632, 1992.

Welsh, K.A., Butters, N., Hughes, J.P., Mohs, R.C. and Heyman, A. Detection and staging of dementia in Alzheimer's disease: Use of the neuropsychological measures developed for the consortium to establish a registry for Alzheimer's disease. Arch Neurol 49:448-452, 1992.

Powers, W.J., Perlmutter, J.S., Videen, T.O., Herscovitch, P., Griffeth, L.K., Royal, H.D., Siegel, B.A., Morris, J.C. and Berg, L. Blinded clinical evaluation of positron emission tomography for diagnosis of probable Alzheimer's disease. Neurology 42:765-770, 1992.

McKeith, I.G., Perry, R.H., Fairbairn, A.F., Jabeen, S. and Perry, E.K. Operational criteria for senile dementia of Lewy body type (SDLT). Psychol Med 22:911-922, 1992

Morris, J.C. The Clinical Dementia Rating (CDR): Current version and scoring rules. Neurology 43:2412-2414, 1993.

Flicker, C., Ferris, S.H. and Reisberg, B. A longitudinal study of cognitive function in elderly persons with subjective memory complaints. J Am Geriatr Soc 41:1029-1032, 1993.

Berkman, L.F., Seeman, T.E., Albert, M., Blazer, D., Kahn, R., Mohs, R., Finch, C., Schneider, E., Cotman, C., McClearn, G., Nesselroade, J., Featherman, D., Garmezy, N., McKhann, G., Brim, G., Prager, D. and Rowe, J. High, usual and impaired functioning in community-dwelling older men and women: Findings from the MacArthur Foundation Research Network on Successful Aging. J Clin Epidemiol 46:1129-1140, 1993.

Mendez, M.F., Selwood, A., Mastri, A.R. and Frey, W.H.,II Pick's disease versus Alzheimer's disease: A comparison of clinical characteristics. Neurology 43: 289-292, 1993.

Förstl, H., Burns, A., Luthert, P., Cairns, N. and Levy, R. The Lewy-body variant of Alzheimer's disease. Clinical and pathological findings. Br J Psychiatry 162:385-392, 1993.

Morris, J.C., Edland, S., Clark, C., Galasko, D., Koss, E., Mohs, R., Van Belle, G., Fillenbaum, G. and Heyman, A. The Consortium to Establish a Registry for Alzheimer's Disease (CERAD). Part IV. Rates of cognitive change in the longitudinal assessment of probable Alzheimer's disease. Neurology 43:2457-2465, 1993.

Stern, Y., Richards, M., Sano, M. and Mayeux, R. Comparison of cognitive changes in patients with Alzheimer's and Parkinson's disease. Arch Neurol 50:1040-1045, 1993.

Fratiglioni, L., Jorm, A.F., Grut, M., Viitanen, M., Holmén, K., Ahlbom, A. and Winblad, B. Predicting dementia from the mini-mental state examination in an elderly population: The role of education. J Clin Epidemiol 46:281-287, 1993.

Stern, R.G., Mohs, R.C., Davidson, M., Schmeidler, J., Silverman, J., Kramer-Ginsberg, E., Searcey, T., Bierer, L. and Davis, K.L. A longitudinal study of Alzheimer's disease: measurement, rate, and predictors of cognitive deterioration. Am J Psychiatry 151:390-396, 1994.

Terry RD, Katzman R, Bick KL, eds. Alzheimer Disease. New York: Raven Press, 1994.

Storandt M, VandenBos GR, eds. Neuropsychological assessment of dementia and depression in older adults: a clinician's guide. Washington: American Psychological Association, 1994.

Friedman, A. and Barcikowska, M. Dementia in Parkinson's disease. Dementia 5:12-16, 1994.

Marder, K., Tang, M.-X., Cote,L., Stern,Y.,Mayeux,R. The frequency and associated risk factors for dementia in patients with Parkinson's disease. Arch Neurol 52:695-701, 1995

Barber,R., Snowden,J.S., Craufurd,D. Frontotemporal dementia and Alzheimer's disease: Retrospective differentiation using information from informants. J Neurol Neurosurg Psychiatry 59:61-70, 1995.

Gregory CA, Hodges JR: Clinical features of frontal lobe dementia in comparison to Alzheimer's disease. J Neural. Transm. 103 Suppl 47: 103-123, 1996.

Growdon JH, Graefe K, Tennis M, Hayden D, Schoenfeld D, Wray SH: Pupil dilation to tropicamide is not specific for Alzheimer disease. Arch Neurol 54:8-8, 1997.

Geldmacher DS, Whitehouse PJ, Jr.: Differential diagnosis of Alzheimer's disease. Neurology 48 Suppl 6:S2-S9, 1997.

Barnes RC: Telling the diagnosis to patients with Alzheimer's disease - Relatives should act as proxy for patient. Br. Med J. 314:375-376, 1997.

Herholz K: Diagnostic imaging of dementia in the elderly. Arch Gerontol Geriatr 25:5-12, 1997.

Mayeux R, Saunders AM, Shea S, Mirra S, Evans D, Roses AD, Hyman BT, Crain B, Tang MX, Phelps CH, Alzheimer's Dis Ctr Consortium Apolipo: Utility of the apolipoprotein E genotype in the diagnosis of Alzheimer's disease. N Engl J Med. 338:506-511, 1998.

Solomon PR, Hirschoff A, Kelly B, Relin M, Brush M, DeVeaux RD, Pendlebury WW: A 7 minute neurocognitive screening battery highly sensitive to Alzheimer's disease. Arch Neurol 55:349-355, 1998

Gauthier S: Update on diagnostic methods, natural history and outcome variables in Alzheimer's disease. Dementia. 9 Suppl 3:2-7:2-77, 1998

Alzheimers Assoc, Natl Inst Aging: Consensus report of the Working Group on: "Molecular and Biochemical Markers of Alzheimer's Disease". Neurobiol Aging. 19:109-116, 1998.

Clafferty RA, Brown KW, McCabe E: Under half of psychiatrists tell patients their diagnosis of Alzheimer's disease. Br. Med. J 317:603-603, 1998

Clinical and behavioral manifestations, and caregiving

Mace NL, Rabin PV. The 36-Hour Day: a family guide to caring for the person with Alzheimer's Disease, related dementing illnesses, and memory loss in later life. Baltimore: Johns Hopkins University Press, 1981.

Mayeux R, Gurland B, Barrett VW, Kutscher AH, Cote L, Putter ZH eds. Alzheimer's Disease and related disorders: psychosocial issues for the patient, family staff and community. Springfield: Charles C. Thomas, 1988.

Teri, L., Larson, E.B. and Reifler, B.V. Behavioral disturbance in dementia of the Alzheimer type. J Am Geriatr Soc 36:1-6, 1988.

Jenike, M.A. Geriatric Psychiatry and Psychopharmacology: A Clinical Approach. Chicago:Year Book Medical Publishers, 1989.

Devanand, D.P., Sackheim, H.A., Brown, R.P. and et al, A pilot study of haloperidol treatment of psychosis and behavioral disturbance in Alzheimer's Disease. Arch Neurol 46:854-857, 1989.

Dippel RL, Hutton JT, eds. Caring for the Alzheimer patient: a practical guide. Buffalo: Prometheus Books, 1991.

Green, C.R., Mohs, R.C., Schmeidler, J., Aryan, M. and Davis, K.L. Functional decline in Alzheimer's disease: A longitudinal study. J Am Geriatr Soc 41:654-661, 1993.

Alexopoulos, G.S., Young, R.C. and Meyers, B.S. Geriatric depression: Age of onset and dementia. Biol Psychiatry 34:141-145, 1993.

C Bowlby. Therapeutic activities with persons disables by Alzheimer's disease and related disorders. Gaithersburg: Aspen Publishers, 1993.

Sevush, S. and Leve, N. Denial of memory deficit in Alzheimer's disease. Am J Psychiatry 150:748-751, 1993.

Drachman, D.A. and Swearer, J.M. Driving and Alzheimer's disease: The risk of crashes. Neurology 43:2448-2456, 1993.

Coyne, A.C., Reichman, W.E. and Berbig, L.J. The relationship between dementia and elder abuse. Am J Psychiatry 150:643-646, 1993.

Fitz, A.G. and Teri, L. Depression, cognition, and functional ability in patients with Alzheimer's disease. J Am Geriatr Soc 42:186-191, 1994.

Lawlor, B.A., ed. Behavioral Complications in Alzheimer's Disease. Washington: American Psychiatric Press, 1995.

Freedman ML, Freedman DL: Should Alzheimers disease patients be allowed to drive? A medical, legal, and ethical dilemma. J Am Geriatr Soc 44:876-877, 1996.

Levy ML, Cummings JL, Fairbanks LA, Bravi D, Calvani M, Carta A: Longitudinal assessment of symptoms of depression, agitation, and psychosis in 181 patients with Alzheimer's disease. Am J Psychiatry 153:1438-1443, 1996.

Marin DB, Green CR, Schmeidler J, Harvey PD, Lawlor BA, Ryan TM, Aryan M, Davis KL, Mohs RC: Noncognitive disturbances in Alzheimer's disease: Frequency, longitudinal course, and relationship to cognitive symptoms. J Am Geriatr Soc 45:1331-1338, 1997.

Gilley DW, Wilson RS, Beckett LA, Evans DA: Psychotic symptoms and physically aggressive behavior in Alzheimer's disease. J Am Geriatr Soc 45:1074-1079, 1997.

Devanand DP, Jacobs DM, Tang MX, Del Castillo-Castaneda C, Sano M, Marder K, Bell K, Bylsma FW, Brandt J, Albert M, Stern Y: The course of psychopathologic features in mild to moderate Alzheimer disease. Arch Gen Psychiatry 54:257-263, 1997.

Dukoff R, Sunderland T: Durable power of attorney and informed consent with Alzheimer's disease patients: A clinical study. Am J Psychiatry 154:1070-1075, 1997.

ALZHEIMER'S DISEASE

Ernst RL, Hay JW: Economic research on Alzheimer disease: A review of the literature. Alzheimer Dis. Assoc .Disord. 11:135-145, 1997.

Friedland RP: Strategies for driving cessation in Alzheimer disease. Alzheimer Dis. Assoc. Disord. Suppl 1:73-75, 1997.

Haley WE: The family caregiver's role in Alzheimer's disease. Neurology 48 Suppl 6:S25-S29, 1997.

Rabins PV: The caregiver's role in Alzheimer's disease. Dementia. 9 Suppl 3:25-28, 1998.

Victoroff J, Mack WJ, Nielson KA: Psychiatric complications of dementia: Impact on caregivers. Dementia 9:50-55, 1998.

Gori G, Vespa A, Magherini L, Ubezio MC: The day care center for demented people: Organization, programs and evaluation methods. Arch. Gerontol. Geriatr. Suppl 6:241-246, 1998.

Logsdon RG, Teri L, McCurry SM, Gibbons LE, Kukull WA, Larson EB: Wandering: A significant problem among community-residing individuals with Alzheimer's disease. J Gerontol.[B.] 53B:294-299, 1998.

Frisoni GB, Gozzetti A, Bignamini V, Vellas BJ, Berger AK, Bianchetti A, Rozzini R, Trabucchi M: Special care units for dementia in nursing homes: A controlled study of effectiveness. Arch. Gerontol. Geriatr. Suppl 6:215-224:215-22444, 1998.

Ballard C, Grace J, McKeith I, Holmes C: Neuroleptic sensitivity in dementia with Lewy bodies and Alzheimer's disease. Lancet 351:1032-1033, 1998.

Borson S, Raskind MA: Clinical features and pharmacologic treatment of behavioral symptoms of Alzheimer's disease. Neurology 48 Suppl 6:S17-S24, 1997.

Bungener C, Jouvent R, Derouesne C: Affective disturbances in Alzheimer's disease. J Am Geriatr Soc 44:1066-1071, 1996.

Cummings JL, Kaufer D: Neuropsychiatric aspects of Alzheimer's disease: The cholinergic hypothesis revisited. Neurology 47:876-883, 1996.

Treatment

Thal, L.J., Fuld, P.A., Masur, D.M. and Sharpless, N.S. Oral physostigmine and lecithin improve memory in Alzheimer disease. Ann Neurol 13:491-496, 1983.

Mohs, R.C., Davis, B.M., Johns, C.A., Mathe, A.A., Greenwald, B.S., Horvath, T.B. and Davis, K.L. Oral physostigmine treatment of Patients with Alzheimer's Disease. Am J Psychiatry 142:28-33, 1985.

Davis, K.L., Thal, L.J., Gamzu, E.R., Davis, C.S., Woolson, R.F., Gracon, S.I., Drachman, D.A., Schneider, L.S., Whitehouse, P.J., Hoover, T.M., Morris, J.C., Kawas, C.H., Knopman, D.S., Earl, N.L., Kumar, V., Doody, R.S. and Tacrine Collab Study Group, A double-blind, placebo-controlled multicenter study of tacrine for Alzheimer's disease. N Engl J Med 327:1253-1259, 1992.

Han, S.Y., Sweeney, J.E., Bachman, E.S., Schweiger, E.J., Forloni, G., Coyle, J.T., Davis, B.M. and Joullié, M.M. Chemical and pharmacological characterization of galanthamine, an acetylcholinesterase inhibitor, and its derivatives. A potential application in Alzheimer's disease. Eur J Med Chem 27:673-687, 1992.

Khachaturian, Z. Editorial: The five-five, ten-ten plan for Alzheimer's disease. Neurobiol Aging 13:197-198, 1992.

Rogers, J., Kirby, L.C., Hempelman, S.R., Berry, D.L., McGeer, P.L., Kaszniak, A.W., Zalinski, J., Cofield, M., Mansukhani, L., Willson, P. and Kogan, F. Clinical trial of indomethacin in Alzheimer's disease. Neurology 43:1609-1611, 1993.

Aisen PS, Johannessen D, Marin DB: Trazodone for behavioral complications in Alzheimer's disease. Am J Geriatr Psychiatry 1: 349-350, 1993.

Singer C, Jackson J, Moffit M, Blood M, McArthur A, Sack R, Parrot K, Lewy A: Physiologic melatonin administration and sleep-wake cycle in Alzheimer's disease: a pilot study. Sleep Res 23:84, 1994.

Breitner, J.C., Gau, B.A., Welsh, K.A., Plassman, B.L., McDonald, W.M., Helms, M.J. and Anthony, J.C. Inverse association of anti-inflammatory treatments and Alzheimer's disease: initial results of a co-twin control study. Neurology 44:227-232, 1994.

Aisen, P.S. and Davis, K.L. Inflammatory mechanisms in Alzheimer's disease: Implications for therapy. Am J Psychiatry 151:1105-1113, 1994.

Coleman,L.M.,Fowler,L.L.,Williams,M.E. Use of unproven therapies by people with Alzheimer's disease. J Am Geriatr Soc 43:747-750, 1995.

Nitsch RM, Wurtman RJ, Growdon JH: Regulation of APP processing. Potential for the therapeutical reduction of brain amyloid burden. Ann N Y.Acad Sci 777:175-182, 1996.

Aisen PS, Marin D, Altstiel L, Goodwin C, Baruch B, Jacobson R, Ryan T, Davis KL: A pilot study of prednisone in Alzheimer's disease. Dementia 7:201-206, 1996.

Baeckman C, Rose GM, Hoffer BJ, Henry MA, Bartus RT, Friden P, Granholm AC: Systemic administration of a nerve growth factor conjugate reverses age-related cognitive dysfunction and prevents cholinergic neuron atrophy. J Neurosci 16:5437-5442, 1996.

Halliwell B: Antioxidants in human health and disease. Annu Rev 16: 33-50, 1996.

Knusel B, Gao H: Neurotrophins and Alzheimer's disease: Beyond the cholinergic neuron. Life Sci 58:2019-2027, 1996

Rogers SL, Friedhoff LT, Apter JT, Richter RW, Hartford JT, Walshe TM, Baumel B, Linden RD, Kinney FC, Doody RS, Borison RL, Ahem GL: The efficacy and safety of donepezil in patients with Alzheimer's disease: Results of a US multicentre, randomized, double-blind, placebo-controlled trial. Dementia 7:293-303, 1996.

Kawas C, Resnick S, Morrison A, Brookmeyer R, Corrada M, Zonderman A, Bacal C, Lingle DD, Metter E: A prospective study of estrogen replacement therapy and the risk of developing Alzheimer's disease: The Baltimore Longitudinal Study of Aging. Neurology 48:1517-1521, 1997.

Knopman DS, Morris JC: An update on primary drug therapies for Alzheimer disease. Arch Neurol 54:1406-1409, 1997.

Aisen PS, Davis KL: The search for disease-modifying treatment for Alzheimer's disease. Neurology 48 Suppl 6:S35-S41, 1997.

Drachman DA, Leber P: Treatment of Alzheimer's disease - Searching for a brearkthrough, settling for less. N Engl. J M. 336:1245-1247, 1997

Haskell SG, Richardson ED, Horwitz RI: The effect of estrogen replacement therapy on cognitive function in women: A critical review of the literature. J Clin Epidemiol. 50:1249-1264, 1997.

Henderson VW: The epidemiology of estrogen replacement therapy and Alzheimer's disease. Neurology 48 Suppl 7:S27-S35, 1997.

Rabins P, Blacker D, Bland W, Bright-Long L, Cohen E, Katz I, Rovner B, Schneider L, McIntyre JS, Charles SC, Zarin DA, Pincus HA, Altshuler K, Ayres W, Bittker T, Clayton P, Cook I, Egger H, Jaffe S, Miller S, Moench LA, Peele R, Phariss B, Shemo MC: Practice guideline for the treatment of patients with Alzheimer's disease and other dementias of late life. Am J Psychiatry 154 Suppl:1-39, 1997.

Sano M, Ernesto C, Thomas RG, Klauber MR, Schafer K, Grundman M, Woodbury P, Growdon J, Cotman DW, Pfeiffer E, Schneider LS, Thal LJ: A controlled trial of selegiline, alpha-tocopherol, or both as treatment for Alzheimer's disease. N Engl J Med 336:1216-1222, 1997.

Small GW, Rabins PV, Barry PP, Buckholtz NS, DeKosky ST, Ferris SH, Finkel SI, Gwyther LP, Khachaturian ZS, Lebowitz BD, McRae TD, Morris JC, Oakley F, Schneider LS, Streim JE, Sunderland T, Teri LA, Tune LE: Diagnosis and treatment of Alzheimer disease and related disorders - Consensus statement of the American Association for Geriatric Psychiatry, the Alzheimer's Association, and the American Geriatrics Society. JAMA. 278:1363-1371, 1997.

Yamada K, Nitta A, Hasegawa T, Fuji K, Hiramatsu M, Kameyama T, Furukawa Y, Hayashi K, Nabeshima T: Orally active NGF synthesis stimulators: Potential therapeutic agents in Alzheimer's disease. Behav Brain Res 1997.Feb. 83:117-122, 1997.

Barinaga M: Neurodegenerative diseases - Alzheimer's treatments that work now. Science 282:1030-1032, 1998.

Rogers SL, Farlow MR, Doody RS, Mohs R, Friedhoff LT, Albala B, Baumel B, Booker G, Dexter J, Farmer M, Feighner JP, Ferris S, Gordon B, Gorman DG, Hanna G, Harrell LE, Hubbard R, Kennedy J, McCarthy J, Scharre DW, Schaerf F, Schneider L, Seltzer B, Siegal A: A 24-week, double-blind, placebo-controlled trial of donepezil in patients with Alzheimer's disease. Neurology 50:136-145, 1998.

Oken BS, Storzbach DM, Kaye JA: The efficacy of Ginkgo biloba on cognitive function in Alzheimer disease. Arch.Neurol. 55:1409-1415, 1998.

Pennisi E: Does aspirin ward off cancer and Alzheimer's? Science 280: 1192-1192, 1998.

Pitchumoni SS, Doraiswamy PM: Current status of antioxidant therapy for Alzheimer's disease. J Am.Geriatr.Soc. 46:1566-1572, 1998.

Joenhagen ME, Nordberg A, Amberla K, Baeckman L, Ebendal T, Meyerson B, Olson L, Seiger A, Shigeta M, Theodorsson E, Viitanen M, Winblad B, Wahlund LO: Intracerebroventricular infusion of nerve growth factor in three patients with Alzheimer's disease. Dementia. 9:246-257, 1998.

Aisen PS, Pasinetti GM: Glucocorticoids in Alzheimer's disease: the story so far. Drugs Aging 12:1-6, 1998.

Farlow MR, Evans RM: Pharmacologic treatment of cognition in Alzheimer's dementia. Neurology Suppl 1:S36-S44, 1998.

Becker RE, Colliver JA, Markwell SJ, Moriearty PL, Unni LK, Vicari S: Effects of metrifonate on cognitive decline in Alzheimer disease: A double-blind, placebo-controlled, 6-month study. Alzheimer Dis Assoc Disord 12:54-57, 1998.

Cummings JL, Cyrus PA, Bieber F, Mas J, Orazem J, Gulanski B, Metrifonate Study Grp: Metrifonate treatment of the cognitive deficits of Alzheimer's disease. Neurology 50:1214-1221, 1998.

ALZHEIMER'S DISEASE